BASIC GYNECOLOGY – SOME RELATED ISSUES

Edited by **Atef Darwish**

Basic Gynecology – Some Related Issues
Edited by Atef Darwish

Published by InTech

Janeza Trdine 9, 51000 Rijeka, Croatia

Publishing Process Manager Marko Rebrovic

Technical Editor Teodora Smiljanic

Cover Designer InTech Design Team

Additional hard copies can be obtained from orders@intechopen.com

Basic Gynecology – Some Related Issues, Edited by Atef Darwish
p. cm.
ISBN 978-953-51-0166-6

For EU product safety concerns:
IN TECH d.o.o., Prolaz Marije Krucifikse Kozulić 3, 51000 Rijeka, Croatia,
info@intechopen.com or visit our website at intechopen.com.

Meet the editor

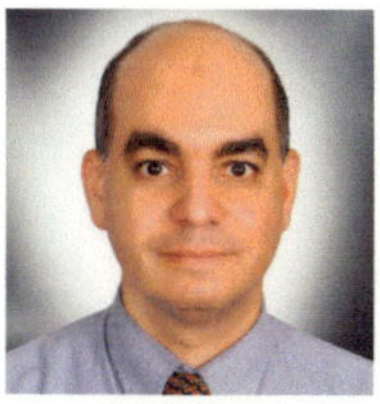

Prof. Atef Darwish graduated from Assiut School of Medicine in 1985 and completed his residency in Obstetrics and Gynecology at Assiut and Ain-Shams universities in 1986-1989. Between 1992-1994, he spent 2 years at the Endoscopic Unit of Ulm University, Germany. Thereafter, he received his Medical Doctorate in 1995 through a combined program between the University of Ulm, Germany and the University of Assiut, Egypt. In 2009, he got a PhD degree in the reproductive medicine at the University of Utrichet, Netherlands. Currently, he is a Professor of Obstetrics and Gynecology, Faculty of Medicine, Assiut University. He authored an internationally registered undergraduate book "Practical Obstetrics and Gynecology" and edited InTech's multi-author book on "Advanced Gynecologic Endoscopy". Prof. Darwish has also published more than 40 papers in international medical journals, and his special interests include: gynecologic laparoscopy and hysteroscopy, reproductive medicine, and assisted reproduction.

Contents

Preface

Gynecology is an expanding specialty that covers a lot of topics. With the rapid and growing advances in all of its subspecialties, the interest of many clinicians in the basic science is declining in their day-to-day practice. Without basic gynecologic science, many gynecologists can't properly understand advanced gynecologic subspecialties. This book is intended to be a study guide for all gynecologists and concentrates on highlighting some basic sciences mainly related to infertility and menstruation. The impact of hyperprolactinemia on women's fertility and health is a very controversial aspect. In this book, you will find detailed explanation of the role of hyperprolactinemia in modern infertility management. Likewise, this book clearly demonstrates the problem of ovarian dysgenesis and best diagnostic approaches. Moreover, a detailed description of a syndrome related to ovarian dysfunction is well addressed. A hint on urogynecology is addressed at the end of this book. Lastly, detailed evaluation of recurrent early abortion is clearly written. In short, this book is tailored to meet the needs of the physicians with different levels of basic gynecologic knowledge. We hope this book would serve as a foundation of valuable information to all gynecologists that they all find useful whatever their subspecialty.

Prof. Atef Darwish
Woman's Health University Hospital,
Assiut University,
Assiut,
Egypt

1

Hyperprolactinemia and Woman's Health

Atef Darwish, Mohammad S. Abdellah and Mahmoud A. AbdelAleem
*Woman's Health University Center, Assiut,
Egypt*

1. Introduction

Background

Hyperprolactinemia (HP) is a real challenge of gynecologic practice. This chapter will cover the following aspects:

Physiologic role of prolactin (PRL) hormone

Galactorrhea

Definition, causes, health problems caused by HP.
Types of prolactin (PRL) hormone.
Estimation of PRL hormone: timing, methodology and factors affecting prolctin level.
Complementary investigations in cases of hyperprolacinemia.

Treatment of HP:

- Health education.
- Pharmacological treatment.
- Herbal preparations.
- New drug delivery systems.
- Choice of a suitable drug for an individual patient.

2. Physiologic role of prolactin (PRL) hormone

The most important of which is to stimulate the mammary glands to produce milk (lactation). Increased serum concentrations of PRL during pregnancy cause enlargement of the mammary glands of the breasts and increases the production of milk. However, the high levels of progesterone during pregnancy act directly on the breasts to stop ejection of milk. It is only when the levels of this hormone fall after childbirth that milk ejection is possible. Sometimes, newborn babies (males as well as females) secrete a milky substance from their nipples. This substance is commonly known as Witch's milk. This is caused by the fetus being affected by PRL circulating in the mother just before birth, and usually stops soon after birth. Another effect is to provide the body with sexual gratification after sexual acts. The hormone represses the effect of dopamine, which is responsible for sexual arousal, thus causing the sexual refractory period. The amount of PRL can be an indicator for the amount of sexual satisfaction and relaxation. On the other hand, high amounts are suspected to be responsible for impotence and loss of libido. PRL has been found to stimulate proliferation of oligodendrocyte precursor cells. These cells differentiate into oligodendrocytes, the cells responsible for the formation of myelin coating on axons in the CNS (Gregg, et al; 2007). PRL possibly contributes to surfactant synthesis of the fetal lungs at the end of pregnancy and immune tolerance of the fetus by the mother during pregnancy (Snyder and Dekowski, 1992). It decreases normal levels of sex hormones (estrogen in women and testosterone in men). PRL, traditionally named from its lactogenic action (mammogenesis and galactopoiesis included), is now recognized from animal - studies to have over 300 identifiable bioactivities corresponding to the wide distribution of PRL receptors, including osmoregulation, reproduction, behavior modification and immune modulation (Bole-Feysot, et al; 1998). 19 Many of these functions are difficult to discern in man, however, where the reproductive roles of PRL are the most evident in terms of clinical disease.

3. Galactorrhea

It refers to the mammary secretion of a milky fluid, which is non-physiologic in that being inappropriate (not immediately related to pregnancy or the needs of a child), persistent, and sometimes excessive. Although usually white or clear, the color may be yellow or even green. In the latter circumstance, local breast disease should be considered. To elicit breast secretion, pressure should be applied to all sections of the breast beginning at the base of the breast and working up toward the nipple. Hormonally induced secretions usually come from multiple duct openings in contrast to pathologic discharge that usually comes from a single duct. A bloody discharge is more typical of cancer. The quantity of secretion is not an important criterion. Amenorrhea does not necessarily accompany galactorrhea, even in the most serious provocative disorders. Any galactorrhea demands evaluation in a nulliparous woman and if at least 12 months have elapsed since the last pregnancy or weaning in a parous woman. Galactorrhea can involve either breasts or just one breast. This recommendation has evolved empirically, knowing that many women have the persistence of galactorrhea for many months after breastfeeding, and therefore the rule is a soft one. The exact numbers have never been established by appropriate studies. Thus, there is room for clinical judgment with this clinical problem. Galactorrhea is present in about 30–80% women; this may reflect the duration of gonadal dysfunction, because women with long-standing estrogen deficiency are less likely to have galactorrhea.

3.1 Galactorrhea with normal PRL level

Only one-third of women with high PRL levels have galactorrhea, probably because the low estrogen environment associated with the amenorrhea prevents a normal response to PRL. Another possible explanation again focuses on the heterogeneity of peptide hormones. PRL circulates in various forms with structural modifications, which are the result of glycosylation, phosphorylation, deletions, and additions. The various forms are associated with varying bioactivity (manifested by galactorrhea) and immunoreactivity (recognition by immunoassay). The predominant variant is little PRL (80-85%), which also has more biologic activity than the larger variants. Therefore, it is not surprising that big PRLs compose the major form of circulating PRL in women with normal menses and minimal galactorrhea (Jackson, et al; 1985).

Simultaneous measurements of PRL by both bioassay and immunoassay reveal discrepancies. At first, differences in PRL were observed based on size, leading to the use of terms such as little, big and the wonderfully sophisticated term big big PRL. Further chemical studies have revealed structural modifications that include glycosylation, phosphorylation and variations in binding and charge. This heterogeneity is the result of many influences at many levels: transcription, translation and peripheral metabolism (Ben-Jonathan, et al; 1996)

Enzymatic cleavage of the PRL molecule yields fragments that may be capable of biologic activity. PRL that has been glycosylated continues to exert activity; differences in the carbohydrate moities can produce differences in biologic activity and immunoreactivity. However, the nonglycosylated form of PRL is the predominant form of PRL secreted into the circulation (Brue, et al; 1992). Modification of PRL also includes phosphorylation, deamination and sulfation.

Most, if not all, variants of PRL are the result of posttranslational modifications. Little PRL probably represents a splicing variant resulting from the proteolytic deletion of amino acids. Big PRL can result from the failure to remove introns; it has little biologic activity and does not cross-react with antibodies to the major form of PRL. The so-called big big variants of PRL are due to separate molecules of PRL binding to each other, either noncovalently or by interchain disulfide bonding. Some of the apparently larger forms of PRL are PRL molecules complexed to binding proteins. High levels of relatively inactive PRL in the absence of a tumor can be due to the creation of macromolecules of PRL by anti-PRL autoantibodies (Hattori and Inagaki, 1997). Overall, big PRL account for somewhere between 10% and 25% of the hyperprolactinemic reported by commercial assays (Smith, et al; 2002).

At any one point of time, the bioactivity (e.g., galactorrhea) and the immunoreactivity (circulating level by immunoassay) of PRL represent the cumulative effect of the family of structural variants despite that immunoassays do not always reflect the biologic situation (e.g., a normal PRL level in women with galactorrhea). Some authors consider women with galactorrhea without HP to have sensitive breasts to trivial stimuli but no evidence supports this postulation.

High blood level (350-400 ng/mL) of PRL composed predominantly of high molecular weight PRL has been reported in a woman with oligomenorrhea and galactorrhea but with no evidence of a pituitary tumor (Jackson, et al; 1985). Big PRLs can also be secreted by pituitary adenomas (Vallette-Kasic, et al; 2002). High levels of relatively inactive PRL in the absence of a tumor can be due to the creation of macromolecules of PRL by anti-PRL autoantibodies (Cook, et al; 1991). Explanations for clinically illogical situations can be found in the variable molecular heterogeneity of the peptide hormones. At any one point in time, the bioactivity and the immunoreactivity of PRL represent the cumulative effect of the circulating family of structural variants. Another illogical situation occurs with large prolactinomas. When clinical and imaging evidence indicates the presence of a large pituitary tumor and PRL levels are low, serial dilutions can reveal very high levels. The falsely low levels are caused by an effect in the assay known as the high-dose hook effect (an extremely large amount of PRL prevents accurate assessment by the antibody in the assay) (Schofl, et al; 2002).

4. Clinical presentations of hyperprolactinemia (HP)

PRL hormone may increase in some physiologic situations that should be considered firstly. They include pregnancy, breast stimulation, breastfeeding, sexual intercourse, stress, exercise, sleep and postictal state. Pathologic HP typically it may cause oligomenorrhea, amenorrhea, galactorrhea, or infertility (Jones, 1995). In hyperprolactinemic women, the incidence of galactorrhea is up to 80%, depending on the diligence with which galactorrhea is sought (Vance and Thorner, 1987). HP may be found in 30% of women with secondary amenorrhea, and in 75% of women with both amenorrhea and galactorrhea (Schlechte, et al; 1980).

It is postulated that PRL acts on hypothalamo-pituitary–ovarian axis. PRL inhibits pulsatile secretion of GnRH and therefore gonadotrophin secretion and has a direct effect on the ovary itself which is supposed to be responsible for the menstrual disturbances that are seen with HP. The amenorrhoea associated with elevated PRL is due to an inhibition of the pulsatile secretion of GnRH. The pituitary gland in these patients responds normally to GnRH or in augmented fashion (perhaps because of increased stores of gonadotrophins), thus indicating that this mechanism of amenorrhoea is a decrease in GnRH (Sauder, et al; 1984). Short-term administration of an opioid antagonist suggests that inhibition is mediated by increased opioid activity (Cook, et al; 1991). However, chronic administration of naltrexone (a long-acting opioid antagonist) does not restore menstrual function (Matera, et al; 1995). Nevertheless, treatment that lowers PRL restores ovarian responsiveness and menstrual function. This is true whether the treatment consists of removal of PRL-secreting tumor or suppression of PRL secretion.

The increase in PRL levels observed in pathological HP results in effects equivalent to those observed during the postpartum period, namely inhibition of the release of GnRH from the hypothalamus and subsequent inhibition of LH and FSH, suppressed gonadal function and promotion of milk formation; this explains why HP is one of the most frequent causes of anovulation.

4.1 Why some women develop menstrual irregularities up to amenorrhea?

High prolactn bioavilability was recorded in women with HP and irregular cycles as well as women with hyperprolactinomas. biological activity of PRL was detected after polyethylene glycol (PEG) precipitation (Kostrzak et al., 2009). Moreover, Macroprolactin (macroprolactin), present in as many as 25% of serum specimens with elevated serum PRL concentrations, can cause apparent HP in the absence of clinical features and lead to unnecessary clinical, laboratory, and neuroradiological workups. Ultrafiltration as well as gel filtration chromatography are effective methods for the estimation of the monomeric PRL concentration of serum thus eliminating macro-PRL interference from PRL immunoassays (Quinn et al., 2006).

4.2 HP in unexplained infertility

Role of PRL estimation in cases with unexplained infertility may have no role except if associated with luteal phase defect (Glazener et al., 1987). It may have a definite role and commonly associated with hypothyroidism in many cases with unexplained infertility (Avasthi Kumkum et al., 2006). Our protocol of management of unexplained infertility is to search for HP in all cases prior to endoscopic evaluation.

4.3 HP and polycystic ovaries

The increased production of PRL observed in patients with PCO is usually transient and does not require treatment (Milewicz, 1984). PCO may be associated in up to 40%. Laparoscopic ovarian drilling may lead to HP in one small sample sized study (Parsanezhad et al., 2005). It is seen in 40% of polycystic ovarian syndrome (PCOS) patients (Conner and Fried, 1998). PCOS and Prolactinoma may co-exist and may need to be treated independently (Bracero and Zacur, 2001).

4.4 HP and sexual function

HP is a common hormonal disorder in women that may affect the phases of female sexual function (FSD). Kadioglu et al (2005) investigated sexual function in patients with HP. A total of 25 women with primary HP and 16 age matched voluntary healthy women who served as the as control group were evaluated with a detailed medical and sexual history, including a female sexual function index (FSFI) questionnaire and the Beck Depression Inventory. Serum PRL, dehydroepiandrosterone sulfate, free testosterone, androstenedione, 17alpha-hydroxyprogesterone, estradiol, free thyroxin and thyrotropin were measured. These variables were compared statistically between the 2 groups. Except for PRL serum hormone levels in women with HP were not different from those in the control group. The median total FSFI score was 23.40 (IQR 17.70 to 27.30) in the hyperprolactinemic group, whereas healthy women had a median total FSFI score of 31.10 (IQR 27.55 to 32.88, $p < 0.0001$). FSD was diagnosed in 22 of 25 patients (88%), while 4 of 16 healthy women (25%) had FSD ($p = 0.03$). Desire ($p = 0.001$), arousal ($p < 0.0001$), lubrication ($p = 0.001$), orgasm ($p = 0.001$), satisfaction ($p = 0.07$) and pain ($p = 0.003$) domain scores were also significantly lower in women with HP. Total FSFI ($p = 0.009$, $r = -0.405$), desire ($p = 0.001$, $r = -0.512$), arousal ($p = 0.002$, $r = -0.466$), orgasm ($p = 0.026$, $r = 0.348$) and satisfaction ($p = 0.041$, $r = -0.320$) scores negatively correlated with mean PRL but not with the other hormones measured. They concluded that a significant percent of women with HP whom we evaluated had sexual dysfunction. No hormonal changes other than PRL and no depression were found as a cause of FSD. We think that these changes could be attributed to anolvulation with subsequent estrogen deprivation.

4.5 Common causes of pathologic HP

Hypothalamic and pitutary causes include Pituitary tumors: micro- or macroprolactinoma, craniopharyngioma, meningioma, dysgerminoma, glioma, chordoma, mixed GH-PRL & adrenocorticotrophic hormone-PRL adenomas, non functioning pituitary adenoma, metastases, hypothalamic stalk interruption, hypophysitis (inflammation), Acromegaly, Cushing's syndrome, Empty Sella syndrome, Rathke's cysts or Infiltrative diseases (tuberculosis, sarcoidosis, histiocytosis X). Medications may induce hyperprolctinemia like Anti-psychotics (phenothiazines, haloperidol, butyrophenones, risperidone, monoamine oxidase inhibitors, fluoxetine, sulpiride), Anti-emetics (metoclopramide, domperidone), Antihypertensives (methyldopa, calcium channel blockers, reserpine), Tricyclic antidepressants (amitriptyline, amoxapine, imperamines), Opiates (morphine, methadone), estrogens and antiandrogens, Verapamil, Protease inhibitors, H_2 antagonists (cimetidine , ranitidine), or Cocaine. Chest wall injury (trauma, surgery, herpes zoster) or spinal cord lesions represent common neurogenic causes. Renal failure or hepatic insufficiency are commonly associated with HP due to disturbed PRL elimination (Melmed, 2001).

4.6 Pituitary prolactin-secreting adenomas

Marked increases in PRL are usually caused by a prolactinoma, a functional adenoma of the lactotroph cells. HP is associated with a PRL-secreting adenoma in almost half of all cases. A markedly high level of PRL (>100 ng/mL) confers a greater risk of having a prolactinoma. It is found in 10-20% of the normal population and account for 25-30% of functioning pituitary tumors identified at autopsy and are the most frequent cause of persistent HP (Mah and Webster, 2002). Probably as many as one-third of patients with secondary amenorrhoea have a pituitary adenoma, and if galactorrhea is also present, half have an abnormal sella turcica (Schlechte, et al; 1980). The clinical symptoms do not always correlate with the PRL level, and patients with normal PRL levels can have pituitary tumors (Speroff, et al; 1979). The highest PRL levels, however, are associated with amenorrhoea, with or without galactorrhea. Prolactinoma is less common in men than in women, typically presenting as an incidental finding on a brain computed tomography (CT) scan or MRI, or with symptoms of tumor mass effect (Kaye, 1996). It is usually associated with markedly increased PRL (>100 ng/mL), but nonfunctioning adenomas and other tumors are sometimes seen with mildly increased PRL. Macro HP should be considered when the PRL is very high, clinical symptoms are mild, and there are no evidence of a prolactinoma. An occasional case has been reported where oligomenorrhoea with Galactorrhea presented with high levels of PRL (350–400 ng/ml) composed of predominantly high molecular weight but with no evidence of pituitary tumor (Vallette-Kasic, et al; 2002). These high levels of relatively inactive PRL, in the absence of a tumor may be due to the creation of macromolecules of PRL by anti-PRL antibodies (Hattori, et al; 1992).

Dopamine-agonists are the treatment of choice of PRL-secreting pituitary adenomas (prolactinomas). Their actions on D2 dopamine receptor (DRD2) and the clinical outcome may be affected by polymorphisms. Prolactinomas are well-differentiated endocrine tumors expressing DRD2. DRD2 polymorphisms correlate with neuropsychiatric disorders, in particular alcoholism and schizophrenia. Some DRD2 polymorphisms, particularly TaqIA, TaqIB and NcoI, are associated with different receptor binding in brain areas. One study carried out on patients with prolactinomas found a correlation between NcoI and TaqIA and resistance to CB. In particular, resistant patients had higher prevalence of NcoI-T allele than the responsive patients, while the commonest haplotype (having TaqIA2 allele) was associated with better response. Only one study was carried out to analyze the role of DRD2 polymorphisms in prolactinomas response to CB. Further studies, including pituitary and hypothalamus in vivo determination of DRD2 binding according to DRD2 genotypes, investigation of possible post-receptorial mechanisms involved, as well as population studies in collaboration with psychiatrists and neurologists, are needed (Filopanti et al., 2010).

4.7 Diagnosis of HP

The diagnosis of HP should be included in the differential diagnosis of female patients presenting with oligomenorrhoea, amenorrhoea, Galactorrhea or infertility or for male patients presenting with sexual dysfunction.

History: Women typically present with a history of oligomenorrhoea, amenorrhoea or infertility which generally results from PRL suppression of GnRH. Galactorrhea is due to the direct physiologic effect of PRL on breast epithelial cells. Pregnancy always should be excluded unless the patient is postmenopausal or has had a hysterectomy. In addition, HP is a normal finding in the postpartum period. Men typically present with complaints of sexual dysfunction, visual problems or headache and are subsequently diagnosed with HP in the evaluation process. PRL suppresses GnRH, causing a decrease in LH and FSH, ultimately leading to decreased serum testosterone levels and hypogonadism (loss of libido, impotence and infertility). Prolactinoma in men also may cause neurological symptoms, particularly visual-field defects. In both sexes, the presence of pituitary tumor may cause visual-field defects, headache, cranial nerve palsies and anterior hypopituitarism (hypoadrenalism and hypothyroidism) especially with macroprolactinomas. Headaches are definitely correlated with the presence of a pituitary adenoma (Strebel, et al; 1986). Although they are usually bifrontal, retro-orbital, or bitemporal, no locations or features are specific for pituitary tumors. Most patients with prolactinoma (the most common type of pituitary adenoma) are women. Most prolactinomas in women are small at the time of diagnosis, and headaches and neurological deficits are rare. Other common conditions to exclude a history of chest wall surgery or trauma, renal failure and cirrhosis (history of alcohol abuse). A drug history is essential because numerous medications have been linked to HP (as mentioned before), usually with PRL levels of less than 100 ng/mL. When drug etiology is suspected, a 1-month trial period off the medicine can be attempted with subsequent remeasurement of serum PRL. Diagnostic challenges can occur in cases when it would be imprudent to stop a medication (i.e., a neuroleptic) and the PRL level is mildly high.

Physical examination: Physical findings most commonly encountered in patients with HP are galactorrhea and occasionally visual-field defects. Visual field Goldman's perimetry is required only in patients in whom tumors are adjacent to or pressing on the optic chiasm, as visualized on MRI. Abdominal examination may give clues for cirrhosis. Generally, HP is discovered in the course of evaluating a patient's presenting complaint (i.e., amenorrhoea, galactorrhea and erectile dysfunction). Typically, the diagnosis is made via the aid of laboratory studies.

4.8 Laboratory serum PRL estimation

In brief, HP is diagnosed when, on more than one occasion under defined conditions, serum levels exceed the upper limit of normal for the particular PRL assay. In the commonly used assays, normal PRL levels in men and women are usually quoted as being <20 µg/L and <25 µg/L, respectively (1 µg/L equivalent to 21.2 mU/L). The defined conditions are a fully awake, fasting individual (for 8-10 hours) with no prior breast or pelvic examination, exercise or sexual activity, in the follicular phase of the menstrual cycle if menses are occurring and is under no significant emotional or physical stress (Zacur, et al; 1997). Plasma levels of PRL demonstrate diurnal variations, where the highest levels are observed during sleep (between 3 am and 9 am) and the lowest levels during waking hours. Thus, PRL secretion is subject to a circadian rhythm and levels should be measured (i.e.; sample should be collected) in the morning (between 9 am and 12 noon) (Biller, et al; 1999). Stress, including nervousness about the blood test can also elevate PRL levels. Mild stress, including the stress of venepuncture, can induce transient elevations in serum PRL, which needs to borne in mind before making a firm diagnosis and proceeding to further investigation. These physiological factors should be taken into consideration in the diagnosis of HP.

Normal levels are typically 10–28 µg/L or <25 µg/L (625 mU/litre) in women and 5–10 µg/L or <20 µg/L (375 mU/litre) in men (1 µg/L equivalent to 21.2 mU/L). However, the reference range for most laboratories is skewed, and a reference range up to 35 µg/L (700 mU/L) may be more appropriate in premenopausal women (Davis, 2004). A mildly increased PRL level (<70 ng/mL) should prompt a repeat test under controlled conditions. Pathological HP should be suspected in patients with a PRL concentration of consistently more than 700–900 mU/litre with no identified physiological or drug cause. PRL levels lower than 100 µg/L may be observed with all causes of HP, while levels exceeding 100 µg/L are usually indicative of a prolactinoma. While the values are certainly not absolute, the recently published guidelines from the Pituitary Society (Casanueva, et al; 2006) suggest that PRL values up to 100 µg/L (2000 mU/L) may be due to psychoactive drugs, estrogens, idiopathic causes or even microprolactinomas, whereas macroprolactinomas are typically associated with levels >25 µg/L (>5000 mU/L). Evidence from a large series suggests that PRL level in non-functioning pituitary adenomas (causing stalk disconnection HP) is almost always <100 µg/L (<2000 mU/L) (Karavitaki, et al; 2006). Levels >1000 ng/ml are associated with locally invasive tumors. Very high PRL levels greater than 2000–3000 ng/ml are probably the result of invasion of cavernous sinuses with release directly into the blood stream. If patients of renal insufficiency take medicines like metoclopramide or methyldopa known to alter the hypothalamic regulation of PRL, PRL levels may rise to over 2000 ng/ml (Hou, et al; 1985). This is based on studies which have shown that levels ≥100 ng/ml are almost diagnostic of PRL microadenoma while the levels between 50 and 100 ng/ml have a 20% risk of having the tumor (Blackwell, et al; 1979). The correct diagnosis can be made using PRL chromatography and polyethylene glycol (PEG) immunoprecipitation (Yuen, et al; 2003). It is more appropriate to employ the PEG precipitation in cases with asymptomatic HP, than repeating measurements of serum PEG level or performing radiological examinations like MRI or CT scan of the pituitary gland as the macroaemia may be the cause but the clinical significance of macroprolactinemia has not been explained yet and is the subject for the future investigations.

Fallacies: Sometimes high levels of relatively inactive PRL in absence of tumor can be due to the creation of macromolecules of PRL by antiPRL autoantibodies (Strachan, et al; 2003). Occasionally in presence of a large pituitary tumor falsely low levels are caused by an effect known as high dose hook effect" where extremely large doses of PRL prevent accurate assessment by antibody assay.

4.9 Other laboratory tests

Pregnancy testing is required unless the patient is post menopausal or has had a hysterectomy. Current TSH assays are very sensitive for detecting hypothyroid conditions. T3, T4 and TSH are done to rule out compensated or primary hypothyroidism. Both of them may be found in cases of HP (elevated TSH with low free T4. Measuring blood urea nitrogen and creatinine is important for detecting renal failure. Patients with macroadenoma should be evaluated for possible hypopituitarism. Initial basal determinations of pituitary and target organ hormones, as well as IGF-1, are measured routinely in order to rule out possible secondary hypoadrenalism and hypothyroidism associated with significant pituitary disease, and to exclude excess GH co-secretion from mammosomatotroph pituitary tumors. Male patients should have testosterone levels checked. Many patients with acromegaly have PRL co-secreted with GH. Anyone thought to have acromegaly should be evaluated with an IGF-1 level measurement and a GTT for nonsuppressible GH levels if needed.

4.10 Radioimaging

Patients with persistent HP should be investigated for possible structural pathology in the hypothalamo-pituitary region, after other common causes have been excluded.

Cone-down view: With newer accurate imaging techniques, cone down lateral view X-ray of sella turcica is no longer the investigation of choice.

CT scanning: When other causes of HP have been excluded, the diagnosis of Prolactinoma is confirmed by gadolinium-enhanced pituitary MRI, though CT with contrast is an alternative. CT scan can detect microadenomas of 2 mm diameter and presence of any suprasellar extension if thin sections and coronal view are obtained. CT scanning (capable of high-resolution 1.5-mm cuts) is able to evaluate the contents of the sella turcica as well as the suprasellar area; however, total accuracy is not achieved (Teasdale, et al; 1986).

MR scanning: MRI is even more sensitive than the CT scan, but it is also more expensive, and it requires a lengthy period of time to obtain the images. MRI provides highly accurate assessments without biologic hazard, and it is better for evaluation of extrasellar extensions and the empty sella turcica (Stein, et al; 1989). Most neuroradiologists and neurosurgeons prefer MRI, as do we. The intention of this workup is to be conscious of cost and to isolate those few patients who require sophisticated but expensive imaging. MR scanning is currently the radiological investigation of choice (Rennert and Doerfler, 2007) because it has a resolution of 1mm and is more sensitive than CT, with the use of gadolinium enhancement increasing the detection of microadenomas. If MRI is contra-indicated or inappropriate, a CT scan with intravenous contrast is the best available option, although frequently repeated scans do entail a significant radiation dose, particularly important with regard to the eyes. Patients with macroadenomas that might impinge on the optic apparatus should undergo formal visual field assessment (e.g. by Goldman perimetry or by computerized charting).

The indications for radio-imaging are:

- Serum PRL level > 100 ng/ml (Bayrak, et al; 2005). However, a recent retrospective study of 104 women with HP suggested that pituitary imaging should be performed in all patients with persistently elevated PRL levels, as pituitary tumors may be observed even in patients with PRL levels just exceeding the normal range (Bayrak, et al; 2005).
- Presence of headaches and visual field defects.
- Abnormal X-ray cone down view of the sella turcica.

With increasing use of these modalities, incidental discovery of pituitary microadenomas is seen in 10% of individuals having normal PRL levels. These tumors are called pituitary incidentalomas (Hall, et al; 1994). Macroadenoma by definition is more than 1 cm and imaging techniques now identify suprasellar extensions, compression of optic chiasma and invasion of cavernous sinus. Therefore, the presence of an MR-scan-detected pituitary adenoma in a patient with HP is suggestive but not absolutely diagnostic that the lesion is a Prolactinoma. On the other hand, no demonstrable lesion may be seen in these patients even on high-resolution imaging, suggesting that they either harbour a microadenoma <2 mm in diameter, or that they have lactotroph hyperplasia or idiopathic 'non-tumoral' HP.

5. Treatment of HP

Goals of treatment of HP

- Elimination of symptoms like galactorrhea and amenorrhoea.
- Induction of ovulation.
- Treatment of PRL secreting macroadenomas.

Recognized indications for therapy include hypogonadism (oligo-/amenorrhoea, infertility, impotence, osteoporosis/osteopenia), tumor mass effect, and significant or troublesome Galactorrhea (Colao, et al; 1998).

Prior to any pharmacological intervention, it is essential to exclude potential physiological or pharmacological causes of HP. The preferred treatment for patients with secondary causes of elevated PRL may be to remove the relevant stimuli. For example, this may involve suspension of a particular medication or measures to reduce stress levels (Biller, et al; 1999).

Treatment options of HP

- Expectant management.
- Medical treatment.
- Surgical intervention.
- Radiotherapy.

5.1 Expectant management

Where no tumor is seen on imaging and there is absence of symptoms like galactorrhea, infertility, menstrual disturbance or hypestrogenism one can use the expectant line of management with serial monitoring of PRL levels and a CT scan every 2 years. Asymptomatic patients may not require treatment (Webster, 1999) and periodic observation should then suffice. Studies examining the natural history of untreated microprolactinomas have shown that significant growth of these tumors is uncommon (Whitaker, et al; 1983). Women with HP but normal regular menses are not at risk of osteoporosis and, again, periodic observation should suffice (Davis, 2004).

5.2 Medical treatment

Medical treatment of HP is recommended to restore menses in young, amenorrheic women concerned about bone loss or to initiate ovulation in anovulatory hyperprolactinemic women who desire to conceive. When symptoms are present, medical therapy is the treatment of choice. Medical therapy affords the greatest benefit to risk ratio and is generally considered the primary therapy of choice when some intervention is warranted.

Indications for medical treatment in women who do not wish to become pregnant include induction of normal menstrual cycles and prevention of potential long-term complications, such as bone loss. Normal conception can occur in some patients and HP is not a reliable contraceptive; oral contraceptives can be given safely to women with HP as these agents do not affect the growth of microadenomas (Testa, et al; 1998). Hormone replacement therapy may be considered in patients with HP-induced amenorrhoea as a means to reduce the risk of bone loss (Franks, et al; 1983). Patients on medications that cause HP should have them withdrawn if possible. Patients with hypothyroidism should be given thyroid hormone replacement therapy. In cases of HP due to psychoactive medications, it is considered unwise to initiate DA therapy for the fear of precipitating a psychotic crisis (Peter, et al; 1993). In most such situations, the exclusion of any significant co-existing hypothalamo-pituitary structural lesion is necessary. Occasionally, psychiatric management can be adjusted and drugs substituted, for example olanzapine, which is said to have a lesser effect on PRL secretion (Karagianis and Baksh, 2003).

The approach to Prolactinomas has changed in the last 25 years, thanks to availability of dopaminergic drugs, characterized by a potent PRL inhibitory effect, a tumor-shrinking effect associated with a satisfactory tolerability. It is considered as the main stay of treatment.

5.2.1 Dopamine treatment

Interestingly, the discovery of a human PRL molecule resulted in the detection of specific reproductive endocrine disorders (e.g., galactorrhea and amenorrhoea), and this event occurred simultaneously with the discovery of a very specific drug capable of lowering PRL levels. From animal experiments performed in the late 1960s and early 1970s, dopamine inhibition of pituitary PRL secretion was suspected (Zacur, et al; 1976). In the 1950s Shelesnyak demonstrated that implantation in the rat could be inhibited by ergot alkaloids, and this action could be reversed with concomitant administration of either progesterone or PRL (Shelesnyak, 1958). It was then shown that this effect could be observed with the ergot alkaloid, ergonovine, and that its action took place at that level of the pituitary gland (Zeilmaker and Carslen, 1962). This resulted in the development by Sandoz Pharmaceuticals (Basel, Switzerland) of 2-Br-alpha-ergocryptine mesylate, also known as CB-154, BC mesylate, or Parlodel. BC was soon found to be effective in the treatment of galactorrhea (Besser, et al; 1972) and to inhibit PRL secretion in men (Del Pozo, et al; 1972).

Dopamine is an endogenous ligand for PRL-secreting cells, binding to cell surface dopamine receptors. Dopamine receptors have been classified into D1 and D2 subtypes, based upon physiological or biochemical responses (Levey, et al; 1993). To date, five dopamine receptor subtypes have been identified, either D1-type (D1 and D5; also known as D1A and D1B) or D2-type (D2, D3 and D4; also known as D2A, D2B and D2C) (Melmed, 1997). Dopamine receptors are located both centrally and peripherally: both D1 and D2 receptors are located in the substantia nigra and striatum, limbic cortex and associated structures (Levey, et al; 1993); D2 receptors are found on the cell surface of lactotroph cells (Schoors, et al; 1991). Peripherally, D1 receptors are located in blood vessels and the proximal tubule cells (Jose, et al; 1998); D2 receptors are found in sympathetic nerve terminals (Mannelli, et al; 1997). The location of specific D1 and D2 receptors has therapeutic implications; selective drugs that act predominantly on one subtype would be anticipated to be associated with fewer side effects than DAs that act on both D1 and D2 receptors. Binding of DAs to dopamine D2 receptors on the surface of lactotroph cells reduces AC activity and inhibits PRL secretion (Melmed, 1997). Several DA therapies are available for the treatment of HP and are outlined in the following table (Hutchinson and Zacur, 1997):

	Bromocriptine (BC)	Cabergoline (Dustinex)	Quinagolide (Norprolac®)
Dopamine receptor target sites	D1 and D2	D1 (low affinity) and D2 (high affinity)	D2
Duration of action	8–12 h	7–14 days	24 h
Half-life (hours)	3.3	65	22
Available doses	1.0 and 2.5 mg scored tablets; 5 and 10 mg capsules	0.5 mg scored tablets	25, 50, 75 and 150 µg tablets
Typical dose	2.5 mg/day in divided doses	0.5 mg/week or twice-weekly	75 µg/day
Dosing regimens, starter packs, dosage	Start on 1.25–2.5 mg/day at bedtime. Gradually increase to a median of 5.0–7.5 mg/day and a maximum of 15–20 mg/day	Start at 0.25–0.5 mg twice-weekly. Adjust by 0.25 mg twice-weekly up to 1 mg twice-weekly every 2–4 months according to serum PRL levels	Start at 25 µg/day. Increase over 1 week up to 75 µg/day. Starter pack (3× 25 µg tablets + 3× 50 µg tablets) allows quick and convenient titration
Advantages	Long history of use; does not appear to be teratogenic (Czeizel, et al; 1989); inexpensive	Good efficacy; low frequency of adverse events; may be useful in BC-resistant patients (Ferrari, et al; 1997); weekly or twice-weekly dose	Good efficacy and tolerability (Webster, 1996); once-daily dosing; simple titration; pituitary selective; use to the time of confirmed pregnancy
Disadvantages	Tolerance; recurrence (Van't Verlaat and Croughs, 1991); resistance; multiple daily dosing	Not yet indicated for use during pregnancy	Not currently available in the USA or Japan
Contraindications	Documented hypersensitivity; ischemic heart disease, uncontrolled hypertension, peripheral vascular disorders; breastfeeding	Documented hypersensitivity; ischemic heart disease, uncontrolled hypertension, peripheral vascular disorders; breastfeeding	Documented hypersensitivity; decreased kidney or liver function
Precautions	Caution in renal or hepatic disease; generally stopped during pregnancy but can be restarted if symptoms recur; perform regular visual-field testing during	Caution in renal or hepatic disease; generally stopped during pregnancy but can be restarted if symptoms recur; perform regular visual-field testing during pregnancy to monitor for	May cause dizziness or hypotension

	Bromocriptine (BC)	Cabergoline (Dustinex)	Quinagolide (Norprolac®)
	pregnancy to monitor for tumor growth; should be given to minimize postural hypotension or nausea	tumor growth; should be given to minimize postural hypotension or nausea	
Interactions	Toxicity may increase with ergot alkaloids; amitriptyline, butyrophenones, impiramine, methyldopa, phenothiazines and reserpine may decrease effects	Toxicity may increase with ergot alkaloids; amitriptyline, butyrophenones, impiramine, methyldopa, phenothiazines and reserpine may decrease effects	Not established
Pregnancy	Usually safe but benefits must outweigh the risks	Usually safe but benefits must outweigh the risks	
Common side effects	Nausea, headache, dizziness, abdominal pain, syncope, orthostatic hypotension, fatigue	Milder and less frequent compared with BC	Milder and less frequent compared with BC (Rohmer, et al; 2000)

DAs play a major role in the management of both idiopathic/non-tumoral and prolactinoma-related PRL excess. These agents act on dopamine D2-type receptors on pituitary lactotroph cells, resulting in a decrease in synthesis and release of PRL (Vallar, et al; 1988). By mechanisms yet to be fully understood, DA therapy is known to cause marked and sometimes dramatic reductions in prolactinoma tumor volume (Webster, 1999).

The majority of medications used to treat PRL disorders are ergot-derived, quinagolide only is not ergot-derived. While all three lower serum PRL on oral administration and also reduce tumor size, they differ in their affinity for D2 receptors and plasma half-life. CAB has the highest affinity and greatest selectivity for D2 receptors. The half-lives of CAB, quinagolide and BC are 65 h (Rains, et al; 1995), approximately 24 h and 8–12 h, respectively, thereby influencing the dosing regimen. A study of 85 patients with macroadenomas, 65 of whom had received previous DA therapy, found that PRL normalized in 61.2%, and a decrease of at least 75% of pretreatment levels was seen in another 28.2% (Ferrari, et al; 1997). Menses resumed in 79.5% of premenopausal patients. Only 4.7% of patients discontinued therapy due to adverse events. Other DAs are lysuride, terguride and metergoline are available.

5.2.2 Bromocriptine

BC ((2-bromo-α-ergocryptine) mesylate) was developed in the 1970s as the first of the DAs to be introduced for pituitary disease, and there is a wealth of data regarding its safety and efficacy (Molitch, et al; 1985) in addition to clinical experience. It is a lysergic acid derivative with a bromine substitute at position 2 (Vance, et al; 1984). The ergot-derivative, BC, stimulates D2-type dopamine receptors on lactotroph cells of the anterior pituitary to reduce PRL secretion (Factor, 1999). However, BC is also able to both antagonize and stimulate D1-

type receptors, resulting in mild adrenal side effects (Bankowski and Zacur, 2003). BC has the longest history of use for the treatment of HP and is well established as a safe and effective therapy (Essais, et al; 2002). Its serum levels peak after 3 h of administration and nadir is at 7 h with very little BC detectable in the circulation after 11–14 h (Molitch, 2001). The biological activity parallels the serum level, but there is continued biological effect even with undetectable serum level. PRL-secreting tumors do not have inactivating mutations in the dopamine receptor gene; thus, DAs can bind and exert inhibitory activity (Friedman, et al; 1994). The oral dose that suppresses PRL is 10 times lower than that which improves the symptoms of Parkinson's disease.

Dosage:

1. Orally:
- Therapy is begun at a low dose (1.25 mg) at bed time with a snack then the dose is typically increased (Brue, et al; 1992).
- It is available as the methane-sulfonate (mesylate) in 2.5 mg tablets. Tablet of 2.5 mg given in a twice daily dose over the course of several weeks as half-life is 8-12 hours. It can be increased to 10 mg/day.
- Slow release oral preparation is also available to be given once a day in a dose of 5 to 15 mg/day and is equally effective with the same side effects, severity and prevalence (Brue, et al; 1992). It is slowly absorbed by the gastrointestinal tract due to the creation of a special capsule. A single oral dose of this preparation can suppress PRL levels for 24 hours (Weingrill, et al; 1992).
2. Long acting depot intravenous injection:
   They are made by embedding glucose initiated polyglycolide microspherules and have a maximum degradation time of 3 months (Espinos, et al; 1994). They are given in a dose of 50 to 75 mg/month. Since response to these injections is rapid they are useful in large tumors with visual field impairment (Beckers, et al; 1992). It has the same severity of side effects as the oral preparation (Brue, et al; 1992).
3. Intravaginal
   It is given in a similar dose of 5 to 10 mg/day. Since it avoids direct contact with the intestinal mucosa it has lesser side effects than oral administration although it provides excellent clinical results (Katz, et al; 1989). So it can be tried when side effects are not tolerated (Ricci, et al; 2001). The levels are sustained for a longer time as it escapes the liver first pass effect when given vaginally and therapeutic results are achieved at a lower dose.

A challenging clinical situation arises when a macroadenoma undergoes symptomatic enlargement during pregnancy. The rationale for using BC during pregnancy for a symptomatic macroadenoma is that:

1. BC shrinks macroadenomas in nonpregnant patients and,
2. The fetal and maternal risks of BC are probably less than the risks of transsphenoidal surgery.

The evidence to support the use of BC for a symptomatic macroadenoma is limited to case reports. The manufacturer of BC collected a series of case reports (Weil, 1986) in which BC was reinstituted after a macroadenoma became symptomatic or used continuously throughout pregnancy. BC was effective at controlling symptoms and preventing the need for surgery in 44 of 46 patients in whom it was restarted for increasing symptoms attributable to a macroadenoma.

Results

There is no question that macroadenomas will regress with BC treatment (Essais, et al; 2002). In 22 clinical trials with BC, in addition to ameliorating the clinical symptoms of HP (amenorrhoea, Galactorrhea or hypogonadism) in 80% of patients with HP but no demonstrable tumors (Cuellar, 1980), these patients had restored menses. The average treatment time to the initiation of menses was 5.7 weeks. BC is known to normalize PRL levels in 80–90% of patients with microprolactinomas (Jeffcoate, et al; 1996) and nearly 70% of those with macroprolactinomas, together with tumor shrinkage (Bevan, et al; 1992).

The availability of BC to reduce tumor size in humans was initially reported by Corenblum and his colleagues (Corenblum, et al; 1975). Since then, of 248 patients reported in 21 series, 76% had some tumor size decrease in response to BC with period of observation ranging from 6 weeks to more than 10 years (Molitch, 2001). Eight series totaling 112 patients quantified the tumor size reduction as well as finding that 45 patients (40.2%) had a greater than 50% reduction in tumor size, 32 (28.6%) a 25–50% reduction in tumor size, 14 (12.5%) a less than 25% reduction, and 21 (18.7%) no evidence of any reduction in tumors.

In a multicentre study of 29 patients with macroprolactinomas, BC successfully normalized serum PRL levels in 27 patients over a mean period of 6 months and reduced tumor size by more than half in 62% of patients (Essais, et al; 2002). In a study investigating the treatment of PRL-secreting microprolactinomas, BC treatment reduced PRL levels in all of the 36 female patients (Moriondo, et al; 1985). A retrospective study that evaluated the long-term effects of BC on PRL levels and pituitary size concluded that BC treatment of mild HP was effective after 9 years of follow up (Touraine, et al; 2001). Since it is highly genericized, BC is an inexpensive treatment for HP. BC causes regression of macroadenomas. In some shrinkage is seen even with low dose (5-7.5 mg/day) while in others large doses and prolonged duration may be required. Usually a dose of more than 10 mg is ineffective (Mori, et al; 1985). Visual improvement occurs within days and tumor shrinkage occurs in several days to 6 weeks, but in some cases it is not observed until 6 months or more. In most cases, reduction in tumor size can take place in several days to 6 weeks, rapid shrinkage occurs rapidly in first 3 months of therapy followed by slower reduction but in some cases it is not observed until 6 months or more (up to 2-3 years) (Mori, et al; 1985). Locally invasive tumors with levels of BC more than 1000 ng/ml show a good response to medical treatment. Problem with treatment of the tumor with this drug is that it has to be taken indefinitely. Indeed, surgical results with invasive tumors are so poor that long-term control with a DA is recommended. After 2 years therapy 75% of microadenomas and 80 to 90% of macroadenomas regress. On discontinuation of drug after 5 years only 25% patients remained normoprolactinemic (Webster, 2000).

Although tumor shrinkage is always preceded by a decrease in PRL levels, the overall response cannot be predicted by basal PRL levels, the absolute relative fall in PRL or even the attainment of normal PRL levels. Visual impairment improves rapidly, but maximal effect may take several months. However, a PRL level non-responder will be a tumor size non-responder. The response of macroadenomas to BC is impressive and a most compelling reason in favour of its use is that it has been successful when previous surgery or radiation has failed (Corenblum, et al; 1975). BC causes not only a reduction in size of individual cells but also necrosis of the cells with replacement fibrosis (Mori, et al; 1985). Although improvement in sellar imaging occurs in some cases, however, the occurrence of spontaneous regression of PRL-secreting tumors makes it impossible to attribute cures to BC. There was 75% reduction in breast secretion by 6.4 weeks and galactorrhea was suppressed in 50-60% of patients by 12.7 weeks. It is important to advise patients that the cessation of galactorrhea is a slower and less certain response than restoration of ovulation and menses. Ovulation was restored within 5 to 6 weeks. Studies have shown successful ovulation induction and pregnancy with BC in the absence of galactorrhea or HP in previous nonresponders to clomiphin (Porcile, et al; 1990). Pregnancies that result from BC therapy do not appear to be at increased teratogenic risk (Czeizel, et al; 1989), even though BC crosses the placenta and lowers fetal PRL concentrations (Bigazzi, et al; 1979). Nevertheless, it is recommended that BC treatment be stopped when pregnancy is diagnosed to avoid potential risks to fetal neural development. Cessation of BC use during early pregnancy does not appear to increase the risk for spontaneous abortions (Turkalj, et al; 1982).

Side effects

However, while BC has been shown to be effective in the treatment of both micro- and macroprolactinomas, approximately 12% of patients experience adverse events even at low doses of BC; these patients are considered BC intolerant (Webster, et al; 1994). However, nearly 60% of patients develop side-effects (Ho and Thorner, 1988), mainly gastrointestinal (nausea, dyspepsia, abdominal pain). Other common problems include postural hypotension, dizziness, headache and faintness. The faintness is due to orthostatic hypotension which can be attributed to relaxation of smooth muscles in the splanchnic and renal bed as well as inhibition of transmitter release at noradrenergic nerve endings and central inhibition of sympathetic activity. Neuropsychiatric symptoms, occasionally with hallucinations, occur in less than 1% of patients. This may be due to hydrolysis of the lysergic acid part of the molecule. 10% patients show these intolerable side effects:

- Immediate effects:
  Nausea, headache, fatigue, dizziness, orthostatic hypotension, nasal congestion, vomiting, abdominal cramps and hallucinations.
- Long term effects (Soule and Jacob, 1995):
  Raynaud's phenomenon, constipation and psychiatric changes specially aggression.

To minimize these side effects we have to build tolerance by slowly increasing the dose (2.5 mg) at weekly intervals, instruct the patients to take the drug at bedtime, individualize the dosage schedule and use intravaginal route. It may help to take the tablet with a glass of milk and snack. The peak levels are achieved after 2 hours and the biologic half-life is about 3 hours. If intolerance occurs with this initial dose, then the tablet should be cut in half, and an even slower program should be followed. Usually a week after the initial dose, the second 2.5 mg dose can be added at breakfast or lunch. Patients who are extremely sensitive to the drug should be instructed to divide the tablets and to devise their own schedule of increasing dosage in order to achieve tolerance. A very small percentage of patients cannot tolerate any dosage.

One 2.5-mg tablet is inserted high into the vagina at bedtime. This dose provides excellent clinical results and few side effects (Ginsburg, et al; 1992). In contrast to oral BC, which is not absorbed completely and that which is absorbed is largely metabolized in the first pass through the liver, vaginal absorption is nearly complete, and avoidance of the liver first-pass effect (with longer maintenance of systemic levels) allows achievement of therapeutic results at a lower dose.

Because many patients with hyperprolactinemic anovulation require treatment to become pregnant, there is a large body of evidence on the fetal effect of first-trimester exposure to BC. There are two BC treatment methods to follow in those patients seeking pregnancy. The first is simply daily administration of 2.5 mg twice daily until the patient is pregnant as judged by the basal body temperature chart. In the second method, BC is administered during the follicular phase, and the drug is stopped when a basal body temperature rise indicates that ovulation has occurred, thus avoiding high drug levels early in pregnancy. The drug is resumed at menses when it is apparent the patient is not pregnant. No comparative study has been performed to tell us whether the follicular phase only method is as effective as the daily method. Furthermore, there has been no evidence that BC ingestion during early pregnancy is harmful to the fetus (Weil, 1986).

No adverse effect of BC has as yet been seen in early pregnancy (Turkalj, et al; 1982). They reported on the results of a surveillance project conducted by manufacturer of BC. Information was gathered on 1410 pregnancies in 1335 women. BC was stopped when the pregnancy was recognized, which typically occurred before 8 weeks of gestation. The incidence rates of spontaneous abortions (11.1%), ectopic pregnancies (0.9%), minor malformations (2.5%) and major malformations (1.0%) were low and not different from the expected complication rate in an unselected population.

The safety of BC exposure in utero has been evaluated by extensive monitoring including multi-centre study of 2587 pregnancies in 2437 women exposed to BC during part or all of gestation, with examination of offspring up to the age of 9 years. Although BC treatment profoundly lowers the maternal and foetal blood levels of PRL (Molitch, 1985), the drug does not appear to be associated with any increase in the risk of spontaneous abortion, congenital abnormalities, or multiple pregnancies and no adverse effects on postnatal development have been detected (Webster, 1996). Long-term follow-up studies of 64 children between the age of 6 months and 9 years, whose mothers took BC in this fashion, have shown no ill effect (Molitch, 2001). Although experience is limited to just over 100 women, no abnormalities were noted with the use of BC through out gestation except in one infant with an undescended testicle and one with talipes deformity (Molitch, 2001).

Nevertheless, because these data are relatively sparse as compared to data in over 6000 pregnancies with BC, BC is favored when fertility is the major reason for treatment. If BC is used to achieve pregnancy, it is stopped when pregnancy is confirmed. With this protocol, the risk of fetal malformation is no higher than the background risk. Patients using BC for infertility should undergo frequent evaluation for pregnancy to minimize fetal exposure to BC. Interestingly, some women restore cyclic menses after pregnancy. This spontaneous improvement may be due to tumor infarction brought about by the expansion and shrinkage during and after pregnancy and there may be a correction of hypothalamic dysfunction followed by disappearance of the associated pituitary hyperplasia.

Disadvantages of BC

- Recurrence:

Recurrence of symptoms occurred in 75% of patients with prolactinomas within 4 to 6 weeks on stopping of the drug. Amenorrhoea recurred in 41% of the patients within an average of 4.4 weeks of discontinuing treatment; galactorrhea recurred in 69% at an average of 6 weeks. Hence these drugs are used only for short-term purpose of achieving pregnancy, curing galactorrhea or reducing tumor mass (Hawkins, 2004).

- Resistance:
  5 to 18% of patients do not tolerate BC or are resistant to it due to decreased dopamine receptor on lactotroph cell membrane. In these cases other drugs can be tried.
- Perivascular fibrosis:
- It may cause perivascular fibrosis in tumors if given for a long time making surgery difficult.

BC has a short half-life (3.3 h), necessitating multiple daily dosing in order to reduce PRL levels. Numerous studies have demonstrated that the less frequent the dosing regimen, the higher the compliance; frequent dosing schedules have been found to reduce patient compliance (Moyle, 2003). Indeed, several studies have demonstrated that compliance with a once-daily dosing regimen can be approximately 73–79%, 69–70% with a twice-daily regimen, 52–65% for a three or 42–51% for a four-times daily regimen (Claxton, et al; 2001). Thus, therapies that offer patients a once-daily dosing regimen would be anticipated to improve patient compliance over therapies such as BC, which require more frequent dosing. In the past 20 years, agents with better side-effect profiles have been developed, notably CAB and quinagolide. Side effects and intolerance with one of these drugs is often solved by using another. A patient who fails to respond to one DA may respond to another.

Although a PRL level nonresponder will be a tumor size nonresponder, about 10% of patients will lower their PRL levels but fail to shrink their tumors (Bevan, et al; 1992). In some cases, the absence of shrinkage is due to cyst formation or tumor infarction. The response of macroadenomas to BC is impressive, and a most compelling reason in favor of its use is that it has been successful when previous surgery or radiation has failed (Bevan, et al; 1992). The problem, however, is that it must be taken indefinitely, because there is yet to be a convincing report of complete disappearance and resolution of tumor that can be attributed to drug therapy and not spontaneous resolution.

Light and electron microscopic, immunohistochemical, and morphometric analyses all indicate that BC causes not only a reduction in the size of individual cells but also necrosis of the cells with replacement fibrosis (Mori, et al; 1985). Nevertheless, PRL levels generally return to an elevated state after discontinuation of the drug. There are cases of improvement in sellar imaging; however, the occurrence of spontaneous regression of PRL-secreting tumors makes it impossible to attribute to BC. Recurrence of HP has been observed after as long as 4-8 years of treatment.

Assiut innovation

During the last decade, we were interested in improving the delivery mode of BC to overcome the common side effects and to increase its efficacy.

Previous work on vaginal BC

In the recent years, research has focused on the vaginal placement of commercial tablets as a logic alternative for patients who cannot tolerate oral treatment. Many studies have demonstrated the superiority of the vaginal over the oral route in terms of dramatic minimization of general and gastrointestinal side effects (Ginsburg et al., 1992, Merola et al., 1991, Merola et al., 1996, Katz et al., 1989). In practice, however, patients find placing orally designed tablets inside the vagina to be inconvenient, a source of local irritation, and a potential hindrance to sexual intercourse.

First innovation: Pluronic-BC combination (Darwish et al., 2005)

In, 2005 we succeeded to add a pluronic to BC to increase its absorption. The aims of this study were to create new formulations of bromocriptine vaginal suppositories that have improved pharmaceutical features and to test their clinical effectiveness and tolerability among hyperprolactinemic patients in comparison with vaginally inserted, commercial bromocriptine tablets. This study had two phases. The pharmaceutical phase was carried out at the Department of Pharmaceutics, Faculty of Pharmacy, Assiut University between May 2001 and August 2002. First, the preparation of vaginal suppositories incorporated 2.5 mg of bromocriptine mesylate (raw material supplied by Novartis Pharma Co., Cairo, Egypt) using a fusion method under ultraclean laboratory conditions. The suppositories were cone shaped, and weighed 1 gram; they were 20 mm in length and 424 mm3 in size. Second, the physical characteristics the suppositories were tested: weight variation, content uniformity, hardness, melting point, liquification time, and disintegration time. Third, in vitro release studies were performed to examine the type of base, partition coefficient of the drug, melting point of the base, hydroxyl number of the base, presence of additives, and concentration of additives. Last, we explored the interaction between the drug and suppository base using differential scanning calorimetry (DSC), and x-ray differactometer infrared spectroscopy (IR). Formulation A included the drug and a base (80% propylene glycol plus 20% polyethylene glycol 20000). Formulation B included Formulation A with solid dispersion with Pluronic F127, prepared by solvent evaporation method. The clinical phase was conducted at the outpatient infertility clinic of Assiut University hospital from September 2002 to August 2003. Fifty-four hyperprolactinemic patients were randomly divided into three groups using 2.5 mg of bromocriptine once daily for 1 month. Formulation A was used by 15 patients (group A), and formulation B was used by 20 patients (group B); commercial vaginal bromocriptine tablets (2.5 mg, Parlodel; Novartis Pharm Co., Cairo, Egypt) were used by 19 patients (group C). The pharmaceutical phase of the study showed an increased dissolution rate of bromocriptine/Pluronic F127 that was 39-fold greater than that of the pure drug alone. First-order release kinetic mechanisms were assessed for formulations A and B. Formula B exhibited a higher release rate constant (k _ 0.51 min_1) than formula A (k _0.048 min_1). The occurrence of in vitro and in vivo agreement can be explained by the presence of non-ion surfactant Pluronic F127. Clinically, most patients entered this study because of intolerance to the oral route (A: 11, 73.4%; B: 17, 85%; and C: 15, 79%, respectively). It was concluded that BC vaginal suppositories containing Pluronic F127 proved to be effective in lowering serum PRL (SP), were well tolerated by most of the patients, had minimal local irritative vaginal effects, and were more convenient for vaginal use than the tablet form.

Second innovation: Rectal approach of BC (Darwish et al., 2007)

Comparison of the rectal and the vaginal administration of the commercial bromocriptine tablets are not published so far. Rectal and vaginal lisuride hydrogen maleates were equally effective in lowering SP if compared with oral administration in a pilot study (Darwish et al., 2005). The pharmaceutical phase revealed that the release pattern of the rectal suppository of bromocriptine mesylate in phosphate buffer pH(7.4) was similar to that of the same formula in citrate buffer (pH 4) which created previously for vaginal use, their release rate constants were 0.60 min-1 and 0.51 min-1 respectively (4). The clinical part of the study comprised 42 female patients with definite high pretreatment SP levels who were randomly classified into two groups. Most of the patients accepted to enter this study due to intolerance to oral route (11(50%) vs. 17(85%)). it is concluded that the approached bromocriptine suppositories containing pluronic F127 were proved to be effective in lowering SP whether used vaginally or rectally. Rectal approach is more effective, has minimal side effects, more convenient for patients who don't accept to manipulate the vagina especially virgins, others fail to use the drug during menstruation, and those patients who believe that the drug may affect their fertility by interfering with sexual relationship. Furthermore, it can be used by intolerant hyperprolactinemic males.

Third innovation: Bioadhesive technology for BC (Darwish et al., 2008)

Transmucosal delivery of therapeutic agents is a popular method because mucous membranes are relatively permeable, allowing for the rapid uptake of a drug into the systemic circulation and avoiding the first pass metabolism. This efficient uptake offers several benefits over other methods of delivery and allows drugs to circumvent some of the body's natural defence mechanisms. Mucoadhesive drug delivery systems are being studied from different angles, including development of novel mucoadhesives, design of the device, mechanisms of mucoadhesion and permeation enhancement. With the influx of a large number of new drug molecules from drug discovery, mucoadhesive drug delivery will play an even more important role in delivering these molecules. We constructed a preliminary study which had two phases. A pharmaceutical phase, which was carried out at the departments of Pharmaceutics, Faculties of Pharmacy, El-Minia and Assiut Universities. It included formulation and evaluation of bioadhesive buccal and vaginal discs containing bromocriptine mesylate 2.5 mg as solid dispersion with pluronic F127 under ultra-clean laboratory conditions. Formulation of Bromocriptine mesylate/Pluronic F-127 solid dispersion passed through the same stages as previously described (7). The row material of bromocriptine mesylate 2.5 mg was kindly supplied by Memphis Co. for Pharm. and Chem. industry, Cairo, Egypt. A unidirectional bilayered buccoadhesive discs were formulated by mixing bromocriptine mesylate/Pluronic F-127 solid dispersion (which is equivalent to 2.5 mg of free bromocriptine mesylate) with bioadhesive polymers carbopol 974P, chitosan and the rest was lactose as a diluent. The mucoadhesive drug-polymer mixture (100 mg) was directly compressed on a previously obtained backing layer of Ethylcellulose (100 mg) using 13 mm diameter die by a hydraulic press machine. A compression force of 2 tones, for 30 sec was found to be satisfactory. The disc is called "unidirectional" because it contains a drug-free backing layer which modifies bromocriptine release towards the mucosa and a drug mucoadhesive layer containing a combination of bioadhesive polymers and bromocriptine mesylate. The prepared discs were of 200 mg total weight, 13 mm in diameter and average thickness of 2 mm. The swelling index, bioadhesion force, surface pH, in-vitro drug release and residence time of the prepared discs were evaluated. These buccoadhesive discs were evaluated for release pattern, swelling capacity, surface pH, mucoadhesion performance, and in vitro permeation of bromocriptine mesylate through buccal membranes. In vivo testing of mucoadhesion time, strength of adhesion, irritation, bitterness due to drug swallowing and disc disintegration in the buccal cavity were performed. On the other hand, vaginal bioadhesive discs of bromocriptine mesylate (single layered) were formed by mixing bromocriptine mesylate/Pluronic F-127 solid dispersion (which is equivalent to 2.5 mg of free bromocriptine mesylate) with bioadhesive polymers including caobopol 974P, chitosan and the rest was lactose as a diluent. The mucoadhesive drug-polymer mixture (100 mg) was directly compressed using 7 mm diameter die by single punch tablet machine. The prepared discs were of 100 mg total weight, 7 mm in diameter and average thickness of 4 mm. The produced discs were evaluated for their swelling behavior, bioadhesion force, in-vitro drug release. The clinical phase was conducted at the out-patient Infertility clinic of Women's Health hospital, Assiut University, from April 2004 to March 2007. Institutional Review Board (IRB) approval was obtained. All patients gave a written consent to participate in this study. In this study, we included all patients with pathologic HP who expressed intolerance or resistance to oral bromocriptine. We excluded patients who received oral PRL-normalizing drugs within at least 2 weeks before the pretreatment blood sample for PRL assay (SP) to ensure complete wash out of the drug. Search for HP was carried out by screening for serum PRL among infertile women with evident galactorrhea, amenorrhea or hypomenorrhea, patients with mastodynea, or infertile patients with sonographic suggestion of HP. Hyperprolactinemic patients (SP more than 20 ng/ml) were randomly divided into 2 groups. Randomization was done by means of a computer program using simple random sample. Neither the subjects nor clinicians involved in the study knew which study treatment was being administered to any given subject. Pharmaceutically, the studied buccal formula gave adequate comfort and compliance during at least 6 hrs. Likewise, tests for swelling, surface pH, in-vitro and in-vivo bioadhesion and in-vitro release expressed satisfactory results. Moreover, it has been shown that mucoadheisve discs containing Chitosan 10% and bromocriptine mesylate/pluronic F-127 solid dispersion expressed a relatively weak in-vivo adhesion (residence time) but when used in combination with Cp 974P (5% w/w) the overall in-vitro and in-vivo adhesions were improved. For vaginal discs, there was no change in the swelling behavior of the discs in pH 4.5 when compared to its swelling in pH 6.8 whereas the release is increased due to rapid disintegration of CS in acidic media. The in-vitro release of bromocriptine from the discs is increased in media pH 4.5 due to the rapid disintegration of chitosan. From this study, we concluded that introduction of bioadhesive technology for bromocriptine mysylate/pluronic F127 administration is valuable in achieving prominent serum PRL reduction in hyperprolactinemic patients in a relatively short duration of therapy. Both buccoadhesive and vaginoadhesive discs are of equal efficacy. Buccoadhesive discs have the advantage of being gender non-specific (i.e. could be used by males), avoidance of manipulating the vagina which is not convenient to some patients like virgins, independence on cyclic estrogen level, and could be used easily during menstruation.

Fourth innovation: Bioadhesive and pluronic F-126 (Darwish et al., 2007)

This study follows the WHO instruction for clinical trials design. The dose of vaginal application is settled in literature as 2.5 mg daily since a long time. This study was preceded by formulation of the drug in a suppository form containing Bromocriptine mesylate 2.87

mg (corresponding to 2.5 mg bromocriptine base) with pluronic F-126 in a special concentration to increase the absorption as a penetration enhancer. Adding Polycarbophil Bioadhasive gel was done which is a polymer that swells in the presence of water. Overall it has a slightly negative ionic charge which produces temporary adhesion to cell surface of the vaginal epithelium. In this study, we included all patients with pathologic HP we expressed intolerance or resistance to oral bromocriptine. We excluded patients who received oral bromocriptine within at least 2 weeks before the pretreatment blood sample for PRL assay to ensure complete wash out of the drug. A pilot phase was carried out on volunteers selected according to strict criteria. The primary endpoints are to assess the effectiveness of the new drug formulation, to investigate the safety including its side effects, and to study the dose-response relationship. It comprised 32 hyperprolactinemic patients who all gave written consent to participate in this study. The study was conducted from March 2004 to August 2004. Search for HP was carried out by screening for serum PRL among infertile women with evident galactorrhea, amenorrhea or hypomenorrhea, patients with mastodynea, or infertile patients with sonographic suggestion of HP. Hyperprolactinemic patients (SP more than 20 ng/ml) were randomly divided into 2 groups. Randomization was done by means of a computer program using simple random sample. Neither the subjects nor clinicians involved in the study know which study treatment is being administered to any given subject. Group A comprised 16 patients who used the new vaginal suppositories once daily for one month. Insertion of the suppository was done by the patient at night before sleep. Group B included 16 patients who used commercial bromocriptine tablets (Parlodel, Novartis Pharma, Egypt) inserted high in the vagina while lying on the back at the bed time once daily for one month. All patients had high pretreatment baseline SP and were advised to take the drug regularly in a fixed time. The patients were instructed to minimize touching nipples and to avoid eating various fowl which contain PRL-releasing factors during the course of therapy. Blood samples were drained from all cases at the start of treatment then every 2 hours thereafter till 16 hours from the start of therapy. Samples were tested for PRL using ELISA method as well as bromocriptine levels using high-performance liquid chromatographic assay of bromocriptine in plasma. Another sample was obtained from all patients at the end of one month of therapy to test for PRL level. Patients were asked to assess their experience with either approach of therapy. In both groups, there was a significant decline of the serum PRL. However, it was more significant in group A. Patient convenience was more evident and local side effects were less in group A than group B in the clinical phase. we conclude that the introduction of bioadhesive technology for bromocriptine mesylate/pluronic F-126 administration is valuable in achieving prominent serum PRL reduction in hyperprolactinemic patients in a relatively short duration of therapy. The formulated vaginal suppositories expressed better convenience with minimal local side effects if compared to vaginally administered commercial bromocriptine tablets. Due to the above demonstrated results, we safely recommend non-use of the commercial bromocriptine tablets for vaginal application.

5.2.3 Cabergoline

CAB is a more recent DA that has a better side effect profile (the most common side effect being headache) with a clinical efficacy similar to that of BC (Colao, et al; 2000). It is an ergot-derived DA (Espinos, et al; 1994) with high affinity for the D2 dopamine receptor (Ferrari, et al; 1986) and, while it can also act upon D1 receptors, it has only a low affinity for these receptors. It is marketed in the US under the trade name Dostinex and received FDA approval in 1996 for the treatment of HP. CAB is a long-acting agonist capable of inhibiting pituitary PRL secretion for at least 7 days after single oral dosing (Cannavò, et al; 1999). Colao and others (Colao, et al; 2003) reported that in 26 patients with macroadenomas, normoprolactinemia was achieved 1 to 6 months after therapy in 21 individuals and after 24 months of therapy in the remaining 5 individuals.

This long-acting agent has a half-life of 65 h, meaning that dosing is performed on a weekly or twice-weekly basis. CAB is dispensed in 0.5 mg scored tablets. It is given in a dose of 0.5 to 3 mg once a week orally or vaginally, usually starting with a lower dose (half a tablet) at bed time with a snack of food. It was given at a dose of 0.25 mg once weekly for the first week, twice weekly during the second week and then 0.5 mg twice weekly. In clinical practice twice-weekly dosing using 0.25 mg is often effective in normalizing the PRL concentration (Verhelst, et al; 1999). CAB dosage in the majority of patients ranged from a total dose of 0.5 to 1.5 mg/wk given in two doses. For patients whose PRL concentrations did not rapidly decline, the dosage range was 1.5 to 7 mg/wk. Dosage changes were made every 2 to 3 months until PRL levels stabilized. After 2 months of treatment, increased doses of CAB were given to normalize PRL levels until a maximum dose of 3.5 mg per week (0.5 mg/day) was reached. In another recent study by Di sarno and his colleges (Di Sarno, et al; 2001) CAB, given up to a maximal dose of 7 mg/wk for 2 years, normalized serum PRL levels in 82% of patients with a macroadenoma and 90% of patients with a microadenoma within 6 months of initiating treatment. Normalization of PRL occurred in 64% of macroadenoma patients and 56% of microadenoma patients treated with BC for 2 years. Pituitary tumor shrinkage correlated with PRL normalization and on average occurred in 80-95% of patients whose PRL levels were normalized. CAB has been found to be better tolerated than BC, and more efficient in normalizing PRL level, improving gonadal function and achieving comparable tumor shrinkage (Di Sarno, et al; 2001). However, it is much more expensive. It normalized PRL and significantly reduced tumor size in the vast majority of patients (Biller, et al; 1996). CAB has been shown in men and women to effectively treat idiopathic HP, microadenomas and macroadenomas that are native to DAs with minimal side effects (Pontikides, et al; 2000). But it is less commonly used in women being treated for hyperPRLaemic infertility, although small case series do not suggest adverse pregnancy outcome (Robert, et al; 1996), despite the fact that this DA has demonstrated a good safety record in the small number (approximately 300) of cases in which it was taken during early pregnancy (Verhelst, et al; 1999). It is useful in BC resistant cases and is more effective in reducing tumor size and PRL levels than BC or quinagolide (Pontikides, et al; 2000).

The low rate of side effects and the once weekly dosage make CAB an attractive choice for initial treatment, replacing BC. Recent data demonstrate that CAB is also effective in treating HP in patients who have failed or were intolerant to treatment with BC (Webster, et al; 1994), which may be explained in part by the longer half-life of CAB, which results in fewer changes in drug concentration in the blood. A multicentre Belgian chart review including 102 males and 353 females with HP treated with CAB demonstrated that CAB normalized PRL levels in 86% of all patients (77% with macroadenomas and 91% with microadenomas or idiopathic HP). Of, these patients, 292 had been treated previously with BC; of these 140 were intolerant and 58 resistant. Tumor shrinkage was seen in 67% and visual fields normalized in 70%. Although 13% of patients experienced side effects only 3.9%

discontinued treatment because of these side effects. To achieve successful results, patients with macroadenomas were found to require higher doses of CAB (1.0 mg/wk vs. 0.5 mg/wk for patients with microadenomas). After CAB, the effects on micro- and macroProlactinomas showed PRL reduction of 95.6% and 87.5% and more than 80% tumor shrinkage in 30.4% and 31.2%, respectively. CAB shrank the microadenomas significantly more than quinagolide (48.6% vs. 26.7%, P = 0.046), but the results are statistically different for macroadenomas (47.0% vs. 26.8%, P = 0.2). In the BC-resistant patients, PRL normalized in 70% compared with 84% of patients with BC intolerance. CAB can also be administered vaginally for the rare patient who cannot tolerate it orally (Motta, et al; 1996).

BC vs. CAB: An evidence based comparison (Nunes et al., 2011)

Cabergoline and bromocriptine are the most used drugs in the treatment of HP, they are able to normalize the PRL levels, restore gonadal function and promote tumor reduction in the majority of patients. A meta-analysis of randomized controlled trials was undertook to compare cabergoline versus bromocriptine in the treatment of patients with idiopathic HP and prolactinomas. The data sources were: Embase, Pubmed, Lilacs and Cochrane Central. The outcome measures were: normalization of PRL secretion, restoration of gonadal function, reduction of tumoral volume, quality of life and adverse drug effects. The meta-analysis of normalization of serum PRL levels and menstruation with return of ovulatory cycle showed a significant difference in favor of cabergoline group (RR 0.67 [CI 95% 0.57, 0.80]) e (RR 0.74 [CI 95% 0.67, 0.83]), respectively. The number of adverse effects was significantly higher in the bromocriptine number than in cabergoline group (RR 1.43 [CI 95% 1.03, 1.98]). The meta-analysis showed new evidence favoring the use of cabergoline in comparison with bromocriptine for the treatment of prolactinomas and idiopathic HP.

Superiority of cabergoline over oral bromocriptine has been proved in many large sample sized studies. A multicentric study on 455 cases done in Belgium proved the high efficacy and tolerability of cabergoline (Vehelst et al., 1999). Nevertheless, this was a non comparative retrospective study of little clinical significance. CSF rhinorrrhea has been reported with both bromocreptine and cabergoline since a long time (Bronstein et al., 2000, Hewage et al., 2000, Netea-Maier et al., 2006).

5.2.4 Quinagolide

Quinagolide (CV205-502) is the other second-generation DA but, unlike either BC or CAB, quinagolide is a non-ergot derived DA with a chemical structure similar to apomorphine. It also provides a safe therapeutic option and higher affinity for the dopamine receptor, so it is efficacious in patients with BC intolerance/resistance (Schultz, et al; 2000). Because it does not act as a D1 receptor antagonist as BC does, it causes fewer side effects and is a better specific D2 DA (Nordmann, et al; 1988). It has a half-life that is intermediate between BC and CAB (22 hours) and is administered daily at bedtime at dosage of 75 to 150 µg/d (Webster, 1996). The dose may be increased up to 300 µg/d.

Although clinically tested in the US, the process of obtaining FDA approval was never completed, so the drug is not available in the US. It is, however, licensed for the treatment of PRL disorders in Europe, where it has been used extensively. Patients in clinical studies who were unable to tolerate BC were better able to tolerate quinagolide treatment (Glasser, et al; 1994).

In women with HP, quinagolide has resulted in an improvement in PRL levels following once-daily treatment with quinagolide with good tolerability (Homburg, et al; 1990) and is effective in reducing pituitary adenoma size and restoring gonadal function and fertility in patients with prolactinomas resistant to treatment with BC (Schultz, et al; 2000). Quinagolide is also effective in decreasing the size of pituitary adenomas (Van der Lely, et al; 1991) and has antidepressant properties (Lappohn, et al; 1992). In an open, randomized crossover trial, quinagolide given as 75 µg daily was compared with CAB given as a 0.5 mg dose twice weekly (Giusti, et al; 1994). CAB users had fewer side effects and PRL levels were suppressed for a longer period of time after cessation of therapy. As a non-ergot derivative, quinagolide is unlikely to cause side effects such as peripheral vasospasm, erythromyalgia, and pleuropulmonary or retroperitoneal fibrosis that occasionally occur with ergot derivatives (Brooks, 2000).

In a study in which 20 women with BC-resistant prolactinomas were treated with quinagolide, normal PRL levels and gonadal function were restored in eight women after 1 year of treatment (Morange, et al; 1996). During a 3-year follow-up period, nine pregnancies were observed in seven women within 1.8 ± 1.5 years (Morange, et al; 1996). Quinagolide therapy was interrupted once pregnancy was confirmed in these women, but was recommenced in two women to control symptoms or tumor growth and was continued throughout pregnancy. All pregnancies led to normal deliveries with no abnormalities noted in the babies (Morange, et al; 1996). In addition, quinagolide has been shown to be more effective and better tolerated than BC (Schultz, et al; 2000).

Quinagolide and BC have been compared in three randomized double-blind studies of 24 to 26 weeks in length with 81 hyperprolactinemic patients. Compiled results demonstrate that 82% of quinagolide-treated patients achieved normal PRL levels, compared with 71% of those who received BC. Only 7% stopped quinagolide for side effects, compared with 23% with BC (Webster, 1996). A randomized controlled crossover trial examined 20 patients treated with either CAB or quinagolide, followed by a washout period with placebo and subsequent treatment with the other of the two drugs (Di Sarno, et al; 2000). Eight of the patients had microadenomas, six empty sella syndromes and six idiopathic HP. In one study, after 12 weeks of the second treatment, a higher percentage of patients (90% of patients) on CAB had normal PRL levels compared with 75% on quinagolide. However, clinical efficacy was similar between treatments in terms of improvements in amenorrhoea, oligomenorrhoea and Galactorrhea. The side effect profiles were not significantly different (De Luis, et al; 2000). Another study reported the treatment of 40 patients with HP or Prolactinomas with quinagolide over 6 years (Nordmann, et al; 1988). Ninety percent of the patients were female, 11 had microadenomas, 12 had macroadenomas and 17 had no radiologic evidence of tumor. Reduction in PRL levels was seen with normalization in 73%, 67% and 82% respectively. The size of the tumor on follow-up imaging was reduced in 55% of the microadenomas and 75% of the macroadenomas. The side effects profile of nausea, vomiting, dizziness and drowsiness was decreased by 75% with quinagolide over BC.

A retrospective evaluation of 11 quinagolide-treated micro- and macroprolactinomas in patients resistant to or intolerant of BC demonstrated an average volume reduction of 46% and 57% respectively (Ilkko, et al; 2002). The average PRL decrease was 65% and 73% respectively. The effectiveness of quinagolide in achieving normal PRL levels in women with macroprolactinomas and HP has been demonstrated to persist after 24 months of treatment (Rasmussen, et al; 1991).

Quinagolide has a 24-h duration of action and this allows for once-daily dosing, which is a major advantage over the multiple daily dosing of BC (Moyle, 2003) and which could offer advantages over twice-weekly CAB in terms of limiting the risk of forgetfulness associated with intermittent dosing regimens. In addition, the 22-h half-life of quinagolide allows this DA to be used until the point of confirmed pregnancy, allowing patients who wish to become pregnant to continue therapy for HP whilst trying to conceive. After the quinagolide treatment, 100% of patients with microprolactinomas had normal PRL levels, as did 87.5% of patients with macroprolactinomas, while tumor volume reduction of greater than 80% was documented in 21.7% of microadenomas and 25% of macroadenomas.

5.2.5 Other DA

5.2.5.1 Pergolide

Pergolide mesylate is another ergot-derived DA that is more potent, longer acting, better tolerated, one-fifth the cost of BC (because it requires only once-daily dosing) and useful in BC resistant patients (Freda, et al; 2000). In one clinical study performed in Europe, once-daily administration of pergolide was shown to be as safe and effective as two- to four-times-daily ingestion of BC (Lamberts and Quik, 1991). This study involved 61 patients (60 women and 1 man) with HP without a pituitary lesion and 96 patients (59 women and 37 men) with pituitary lesions exceeding 5 mm.

Pergolide is given in a single daily dose of 50-150 µg. It was started as a 25 µg dose taken orally with the evening meal for the first 3 days. Dosage was advanced in 25 µg increments every 3 to 4 days until a total dose of 300 µg per day was reached. BC was begun at a 1.25 mg/day oral dose with the evening meal and increased every fourth day in 1.25 to 2.5 mg increments given in divided doses (three per day) in total dosage that did not exceed 20 mg per day and 30 mg per day for the non-pituitary tumor and pituitary tumor groups, respectively. Both drugs were equally effective in lowering PRL levels and were equally effective in shrinking pituitary lesions.

In another study with pergolide, 22 consecutive patients with macroprolactinomas were followed prospectively; an 88% reduction in PRL levels was found with 15 of the 22 normalizing. Mean tumor shrinkage was 50% or greater in 77% of patients and 75% or greater in 45% of patients. Visual abnormalities were reversible after pergolide therapy in all but 1 of 12 patients with abnormal testing (Orrego, et al; 2000). If continued treatment with a DA is needed, another DA should be substituted for Pergolide (Valdemarsson, 2004).

5.2.5.2 Lisuride

It is a dopamine and serotonin receptor partial agonist. It has a high affinity for the dopamine D2, D3 and D4 receptors, as well as serotonin 5-HT1A and 5-HT2A/C receptors. It is used since the 1980s for its prolactin-lowering and anti-Parkinson activity.

It is very effective PRL-normalizing drug with relatively less serious complications if compared to other groups. Unfortunately, oral intolerance is frequently seen among patients up to the level of discontinuation of the drug due to systemic and GIT complications. Its current oral tablet form requires dramatic modification to restore the high tolerability rate. Despite its common side effects, it is superior to other prolactin normalizing drugs in being extremely potent 5-HT(2B) antagonist. Drug-induced cardiac valvulopathies are always related to a stimulatory drug effect on trophic 5-HT(2B) receptors. As lisuride is devoid of such an effect, but on the contrary is an extremely potent 5-HT(2B) antagonist, an association of lisuride therapy with cardiac valvulopathies seems to be highly unlikely. All ergot-derived drugs and especially DA receptor agonists with some chemical similarity to the ergot structure will cause or facilitate cardiac valvulopathies as observed with pergolide (Hofmann et al., 2006).

5.2.5.3 Hydergeine

Hydergeine (ergaloid mesylate) is a mixed ergot alkaloid that has been shown to increase cognitive function in selected patients with neurologic disorders. It is approved only for this purpose in the US. It has, however, been used to treat HP and has been found to lower PRL levels only if serum PRL levels are less than 100 ng/ml. It is well tolerated by patients and should be used in cases where BC fails resulting in pregnancy in some patients (Tamura, et al; 1989).

5.2.5.4 Pramipexole

Pramipexole is a non-ergot DA. It is a derivative of aminobenzathiazole which primarily affects the D2 subfamily of dopamine receptors. Studies investigating the effects of this new DA on PRL secretion in humans are limited. In one small study performed in 1992, pramipexole decreased serum PRL levels in a dose-dependent manner, with a maximum effect after 2 to 4 hours (Schilling, et al; 1992). Side effects from this DA are frequent and similar to those encountered after the use of other DAs and include nausea, insomnia, constipation and orthostatic hypotension.

Response monitoring

Response to therapy should be monitored by checking fasting serum PRL levels and checking tumor size with MRI. Most women (approximately 90%) regain cyclic menstruation and achieve resolution of galactorrhea. Testosterone levels in men increase but may remain below normal. Therapy should be continued for approximately 12-24 months (depending on the degree of symptoms or tumor size) and then withdrawn if PRL levels have returned to the normal range. After withdrawal, approximately one sixth of patients maintain normal PRL levels. Normalization of visual fields is observed in as many as 90% of patients. A failure to improve within 1-3 months is an indication for surgery. Tumors usually shrink to 50% of their original size in approximately 90% of patients treated for macroadenomas for 1 year. In patients with nonProlactinoma tumors (masses that are compressing the pituitary stalk), medical treatment reduces serum PRL levels but does not reduce tumor size. CAB is somewhat more effective than BC in terms of tumor shrinkage (Wilson, 1998).

Compliance

Often, poor patient compliance may mimic apparent primary resistance (Webster, 1996). Non-compliance, defined as any deviation by the patient from a physician's instructions, is associated with treatment failure, resulting in inefficient use of time for the physician and patient and in increased costs of health management (Rizzo and Simons, 1997). Compliance with DAs is important to ensure optimal treatment success. However, BC is associated with features that may reduce compliance, namely a poor side effect profile owing to its non-selective mechanism of action, and a short duration of action that necessitates multiple daily dosing. Approximately 5% of patients terminated treatment because of adverse reactions. The problem is that PRL returns to elevated levels in 75% of patients after discontinuation of treatment with DAs, and there is no clinical or laboratory assessment that can predict those patients who will have a beneficial long-term result (Hawkins, 2004). This is the major reason we use DA treatment only to achieve a specific purpose: pregnancy, suppression of bothersome galactorrhea, or reduction in tumor mass. Both quinagolide and CAB offer patients an improved side effect profile over BC, as well as an improved dosing regimen. Additionally, quinagolide can be used until pregnancy is confirmed and may therefore result in improve compliance in females wishing to become pregnant.

Resistance to DAs

Resistance to DAs in prolactinomas, defined as failure to normalize serum PRL levels and failure to reduce tumor size, is thought to relate to a low density of membrane D2 receptors on some lactotroph tumors (Pellegrini, et al; 1989). A complete lack of response to pharmacotherapy is a rare occurrence, with partial response occurring more frequently. A range of 10–20% of patients does not achieve reductions in PRL levels or tumor size after treatment with DAs, even at high doses (Di Sarno, et al; 2001). There is no consensus on the criteria to define resistance, but some proposed definitions for BC resistance include the following:

- The absence of normalized PRL levels after treatment with 15 µg/day BC for 3 months (Hawkins, 2004).
- A less than 50% reduction in serum PRL levels despite treatment with 15 µg/day BC (Luque, et al; 1986).

Resistance to DAs may be due to reduced number of cell surface dopamine receptors, abnormal post-translational processing of receptors, or abnormal intracellular signaling pathways. Lactotrope heterogeneity, as defined by the difference in response to dopamine by different cell populations of lactotropes, may explain this phenomenon (Luque, et al; 1986). The failure of a tumor to shrink significantly in size despite a normalization of PRL levels can be consistent with a nonfunctioning tumor that is interrupting the supply of dopamine to the pituitary by stalk compression. Early surgery is indicated. A tumor that continues to grow despite DA treatment can be a rare carcinoma.

The cross-tolerability of DAs is unpredictable. Evidence suggests that fewer patients show resistance to CAB compared with BC (Di Sarno, et al; 2001). Ninety-seven percent of patients intolerant to BC tolerated CAB. This proportion is no different from the general population (Webster, 1996). Additionally, quinagolide has shown efficacy in patients resistant to or unable to tolerate BC therapy (Di Sarno, et al; 2000). Thus, both quinagolide and CAB may be used to treat patients with prolactinomas who are resistant or intolerant to treatment with BC (Rohmer, et al; 2000).

Management of DA resistance currently includes progressive increase in the DA dosage, changing the DA, and resorting to trans-sphenoidal pituitary surgery if necessary. A novel class of compounds called PRL resistance antagonists, akin to the GH-receptor antagonist pegvisomant used in acromegaly may have a future therapeutic role in DA-resistant prolactinomas (Goffin, et al; 2006).

Recurrence

Recurrence of HP and re-expansion of previously shrunken pituitary adenomas is a well-known phenomenon after cessation of DA therapy. Few systematic clinical studies have been performed to provide guidance in this area. A comparative study examined 23 patients with microprolactinomas and 16 with macroprolactinomas, all previously intolerant of BC (Hawkins, 2004). Five patients with macroadenomas had also undergone surgery, and one with a microadenoma. All patients received quinagolide for 1 year followed by CAB for 1 year. A washout period after each treatment is performed to evaluate recurrence of HP.

All patients had recurrence of HP within 15 to 60 days of withdrawal of therapy, but post-quinagolide/pre-CAB levels were significantly lower than initial levels in both groups. Withdrawal of CAB led to recurrence of HP in 15 of 23 microprolactinomas and all macroprolactinomas within 30 days. Both drugs were well tolerated. In another study using CAB to treat patient with microadenomas for 12 months, normoprolactinemia was maintained in 4 of 26 patients (18%) 2 months after drug treatment was stopped (Muratori, et al; 1997).

In a more recent study by Passos and his colleges (Passos, et al, 2002) 131 patients (62 with microprolactinoma and 69 with macroprolactinoma) were treated with BC for a median time of 47 months, during which time normalization of PRL levels was observed. After cessation of treatment, normoprolactinemia remained in 26% of the microprolactinoma group when studied and 16% in the macroprolactinoma group for a median time of 44 months. These results are in agreement with other studies that have suggested that the longer the duration of DA therapy, the greater is the chance that normoprolactinemia will be sustained. Long-term DA treatment has been associated with perivascular fibrosis of pituitary adenoma tumor cells (Landolt and Osterwalder, 1984). Subclinical pituitary apoplexy has been observed after pregnancy in women with macroadenomas and during BC therapy.

Dopamine agonists and pregnancy

HP is a frequent cause of anovulatory infertility and luteal phase defect. Dopaminergic treatment is the first line of treatment and is very effective in both idiopathic HP and prolactinoma, with a 60 to 80% pregnancy rate. DAs are normally stopped following confirmation of pregnancy in order to avoid any possible teratogenic risk and so as not to prevent lactation at term. Even when DAs are discontinued early, the fetus is probably exposed to these drugs for up to 3–4 weeks of gestation; however, no adverse outcome has been reported during pregnancy (Krupp and Monka, 1987) or childhood (Raymon, et al; 1985). Whereas BC has a proven safety record in pregnancy (Molitch, 1999), the data on CAB and quinagolide are still limited. DAs impair lactation and hence are avoided in the postpartum period when breastfeeding is desired by the patient.

Owing to the accumulated evidence suggesting that BC does not evoke teratogenic or embryopathic effects in humans, continuation of BC therapy during pregnancy may be considered in cases of macroprolactinoma or where there is evidence of tumor expansion

The therapeutic strategy for pregnant women with macroprolactinomas should be individualized for each patient, considering both the potential effects of a therapy on foetal development and the effects of pregnancy on the prolactinoma. If DA therapy is continued throughout pregnancy, careful follow-up is required, with monthly visual-field examinations and MRI for patients who develop symptoms of tumor enlargement of visual field defects.

As a general principle, fetal exposure to DA should be limited to as short a period as possible. Mechanical contraception should be used until the first two to three cycles have occurred so that an intermenstrual period can be established and the woman will know when she has missed a menstrual period. The DA can be stopped after being given for only 3–4 weeks of gestation. When used in this fashion, BC has not been found to cause any increase in spontaneous abortions, ectopic pregnancies, trophoblastic disease, multiple pregnancies or congenital malformation (Molitch, 2001).

Gradual withdrawal

DA agents are the treatment of choice for macroadenomas, utilizing as low a dose as possible. Once shrinkage has occurred, the daily dose should be progressively reduced until the lowest maintenance dose is achieved. The serum PRL level can be utilized as a marker, checking levels every 3 months until stable. In many (but not all) patients, control of tumor growth correlates with maintenance of a baseline PRL level and can be achieved in some patients with as little as one-quarter of a BC tablet (0.625 mg) daily (Liuzzi, et al; 1985).

Withdrawal of the drug can be associated with regrowth or reexpansion of the tumor, and, therefore, treatment must be at least for several years, many tumors (70-80%) do not regrow (Colao, et al; 2003). If there is a good response in PRL levels, and if present, visual field defects, the MRI should be repeated after 1 year of treatment to establish size reduction of the tumor. If clinician and patient need reassurance regarding tumor size, imaging intervals can be prolonged if the tumor is stable; e.g., at 1 year, 2 years, 4 years, 8 years. It should be noted that progressively increasing PRL levels have been observed without associated tumor growth of a microadenoma (Sisam, et al; 1986). Some patients prefer surgery rather than long-term medical treatment, and it is certainly a legitimate option. In view of better results claimed in more recent times, this choice should be presented to the patient.

Estrogen replacement therapy

When a woman with raised PRL does not wish to become pregnant, intolerant to various DAs or the tumor is small but is producing significant hypestrogenism, estrogen replacement therapy should be given for protection of the bones and vascular system (Jeffcoate, et al; 1996). It is may be warranted to prevent osteoporosis or to improve libido. Hypogonadal women with microprolactinomas may therefore be treated for their hypogonadism with combined oral contraceptive agents (Molitch, 1999) when galactorrhea is not a major problem. When contraception is needed they can be put on low dose contraceptive pills. There is no risk of tumor expansion due to estrogens since the level given is only enough to raise levels up to those in natural cycle (Losa, et al; 2002). While published data on patients with prolactinomas who are treated with oral contraceptives for hypogonadism have not shown any substantial risk for tumor enlargement (Corenblum and

Donovan, 1993), it is advisable to monitor patients who use oral contraceptives carefully with periodic measurement of PRL levels (Garcia and Kapcala, 1995). If ovulation still does not occur in patients with HP following treatment with a DA, attempts can be made to induce ovulation with anti-estrogens, gonadotrophins or pulsatile GnRH administration. If pregnancy does not occur after 6–8 months of ovulatory cycles, the patient must be reinvestigated. Patients who do not wish to conceive should be advised to use contraception, as return of fertility may not be immediately apparent.

5.2.6 Chaste tree berry

Chaste tree (Vitex agnus-castus), also known as monk's pepper, is used in Germany for irregular periods, pre-menstrual pain, and feelings of tension and swelling in the breasts. The purpose of this study was to evaluate the chaste tree berry as a treatment for mild HP and mastalgia and to compare its efficacy with BC, a conventional therapy.

A group of women with cyclic mastalgia (n=40) and a group of women with mild HP (n=40) participated in this prospective, randomized, comparative study. (This Brief Communication does not give additional methodological details.) In each group the patients were randomized to receive either BC (Parlodel® 2.5 mg twice daily, Novartis, Turkey) or chaste tree berry (Agnucaston®, 40 mg daily, Bimeks, Germany) for 3 months. Serum PRL and breast pain were evaluated preand post-treatment.

PRL levels were significantly reduced by both treatments ($P<0.0001$). There was no significant difference in the size of the effect between treatments. Breast pain was significantly less after both treatments ($P<0.0001$), and there was no significant difference between treatments in regard to breast pain. No adverse events associated with chaste tree berry were reported. Thirteen percent of the patients taking BC reported nausea and vomiting.

The results show that chaste tree berry has PRL and breast pain reducing abilities similar to BC. However, chaste tree berry has better patient compliance and lower cost. The authors recommend chaste tree berry as a first-line treatment for cyclic mastalgia and mild HP. Although these results are promising, the group sizes were small and the study should be reconfirmed with a larger number of patients. Furthermore, this trial did not contain a placebo group; therefore, it is not possible to ascertain the magnitude of the placebo effect in this intervention. The lack of a placebo group is additionally problematic given the study design. It is assumed that the mechanism of action for the reduction of mastalgia is the lowering of PRL (via binding dopamine receptors on the pituitary by either agent); however this association is not clarified. The reduction of PRL in both the hyperprolatinaemia group and the cyclic mastlagia group, with the additional reduction in pain in the mastalgia group, while significant, does not prove the association between lowered PRL and decreased mastalgia. The decreased mastalgia could be due to placebo or other unidentified effects. This study has clinical relevance in that the mechanism could elucidate other indications and contraindications to this therapy. Nonetheless, the trial is a compelling look at the effect of chaste tree berry as a treatment alternative for mastalgia (Kilicdag, et al; 2004).

5.3 Surgical intervention

The efficacy of medical treatment in restoring a normoprolactinemic state without the risk of pituitary insufficiency has limited the indications for surgical resection of prolactinomas.

Surgery may achieve a long-term cure, but remission rates are no better than 60% (Colao, et al; 2003). Nowadays, surgery is usually reserved for cases of intolerance/resistance to medical therapy, persistent tumor mass effect despite maximal DA treatment, and considered in patients who are dependent on antipsychotic medication.

Indications for surgery

Transsphenoidal surgery in pregnancy is indicated in certain circumstances. General indications for pituitary surgery include:

- Patient unwilling for long-term drug therapy.
- Intolerable side effects of drugs.
- Tumors resistant to medical therapy.
- Patients who have persistent visual-field defects in spite of medical treatment.
- Patients with large cystic or hemorrhagic tumors.
- Nonfunctioning tumors where PRL levels are not very high. These tumors may expand with invasion into cavernous sinus, compression of optic chiasma and hemorrhage causing pituitary apoplexy.
- Suprasellar extension not regressing with drug therapy.

5.4 Radiotherapy

Because tumor recurrence after surgery is high, radiotherapy should be considered (Tsagarakis, et al; 1991). It is not the primary choice of treatment and may be tried if medical management or surgery fails. It has a role for macroprolactinomas that are not responsive to other modes of treatment, or when medical and/or surgical therapies are contra-indicated/felt to be inappropriate. Irradiation should be reserved as adjunctive therapy for controlling postoperative persistence or regrowth of large tumors and shrinking large tumors that are unresponsive to medical treatment. It is given using linear cobalt or proton mode. Conventional radiation therapy over a period of 5-6 weeks has been observed to decrease tumor size and PRL secretion (Tsang, et al; 1996). More modern radiotherapy strategies, namely gamma knife and focal radiation surgeries have been designed to reduce the radiation exposure of brain structures outside the target area and deliver a higher dose of radiation to the target area to provide more effective therapy in a single treatment session (Tsang, et al; 1996). However, experience with these techniques remains limited at this time and may increase the risk of hypopituitarism.

Clinical conditions deserve special attention

Lymphocytic hypophysitis

It is a rare, autoimmune, inflammatory disorder that is most often associated with pregnancy and can be present in a fashion similar to that of a pituitary adenoma. The etiology of lymphocytic hypophysitis is unknown but is associated with other autoimmune disorders (Feigenbaum, et al; 1991). Histologic features include lymphocytic infiltration of the anterior pituitary with associated destruction and fibrosis of the gland. Radiographic features are non specific and the appearance mimics that of a pituitary adenoma. The clinical symptoms are attributable to a mass effect on adjoining structures: headache, visual disturbances or pituitary dysfunction. There is no unique endocrinologic profile associated with lymphocytic hypophysitis. It can present with HP, diabetes insipidus or hypopituitarism. The diagnosis is made by transsphenoidal biopsy and steroids are the first-line therapy (Kerrison and Lee, 1997).

Empty sella syndrome

A patient may have an abnormal sella turcica, but rather than a tumor, she can have the empty sella syndrome. In this condition, there is a congenital incompleteness of the sellar diaphragm that allows an extension of the subarachnoid space into the pituitary fossa. The pituitary gland is separated from the hypothalamus and is flattened. The empty sella syndrome may develop secondary to surgery, radiotherapy, or infarction of a pituitary tumor. An empty sella is found in approximately 5% of autopsies, and approximately 85% are in women, previously thought to be concentrated in middle-aged and obese women (Hodgson, et al; 1972). A closer look at the sella turcica, brought about by our pursuit of elevated PRL levels, has revealed an incidence of empty sella in 4-16% of patients who present with amenorrhoea/galactorrhea (Schlechte, et al; 1980). Galactorrhea and elevated PRL levels can be seen with an empty sella, and there may be a coexisting PRL-secreting adenoma. This suggests that the empty sella in these patients may have arisen because of tumor infarction. This condition is benign; it does not progress to pituitary failure. The chief hazard to the patient is inadvertent treatment for a pituitary tumor. Because of the possibility of a coexisting adenoma, patients with elevated PRL levels or galactorrhea and an empty sella should undergo annual surveillance (PRL assay and imaging) for a few years to detect tumor growth. It is totally safe and appropriate to offer hormone treatment or induction of ovulation.

Pituitary apoplexy

Hemorrhage or necrosis of a pituitary adenoma is an endocrine emergency. The classic, acute syndrome presents over 1-2 days and is characterized by headache, meningeal signs, visual disturbances and neurologic dysfunction. Recent improvements in MRI technology have revealed a subclinical form of pituitary apoplexy in which a small pituitary hemorrhage causes few symptoms. Patients with pituitary apoplexy require intensive support and treatment for hypopituitarism. Worsening visual disturbances or signs of pituitary compression are indications for transsphenoidal decompression.

Keynote points

- Clinical attention towards hyperprolactinemia starts by proper examination of breasts.
- Think of physiologic causes and medications.
- Hyperprolactinemia may affect women's health indifferent ways.
- Dopamine agonists are highly effective for treating hyperprolactinemic amenorrhea and infertility.
- Bromocriptine is the treatment of choice when pregnancy is the goal.
- Alternative bromocriptine delivery approaches are interesting promising modifications that would minimize side effects and increase efficacy.
- Cabergoline is better tolerated and is effective in patients resistant to bromocriptine, but more studies are needed before it can be recommended as first-line treatment for HP in women wishing to conceive.
- Because microadenomas do not grow progressively larger, long-term treatment isn't necessary to prevent tumor growth.

- In carefully selected women with small tumors, consider prescribing an oral contraceptive instead of a dopamine agonist, when fertility is not an issue (Schlechte J, Goldner W,2004).

6. References

Avasthi Kumkum, Kaur Jasmine, Gupta Shweta, Narang Pal Ajeshwar (2006) Hyperprolactinema and its correlation with hypothyroidism in infertile women intolerant to oral dopaminergics. J Obstet Gynecol India Vol. 56, No. 1, 68-71

Bankowski BJ and Zacur HA. (2003) Dopamine agonist therapy for hyperprolactinemia, Clin Obstet Gynecol 46, pp. 349–362.

Bayrak A, Saadat P, Mor E, Chong L, Paulson RJ, Sokol RZ. (2005) Pituitary imaging is indicated for the evaluation of hyperprolactinaemia. Fertil Steril; 84(1):181-5.

Beckers A, Petrossians P, Abs R, Flandroy P, Stadnik T, de Longueville M, Lancranjan I, Stevenaert A. (1992) Treatment of macroprolactinomas with long acting and repeatable form of bromocriptine: a report of 29 cases. J Clin Endocrinol Metab; 75:275.

Ben-Jonathan N, Mershon JL, Allen DL, Steinmetz RW. (1996) Extrapituitary prolactin: distribution, regulation, functions, and clinical aspects, Endocr Rev 17:639-669.

Besser GM, Parke L, Edwards CR, Forsyth IA, McNeilly AS. (1972) Galactorrhea: successful treatment; with reduction of plasma prolactin levels by bromo-ergocriptine. Br Med J. 3: 669-672.

Bevan JS, Webster J, Burke CW, Scanlon MF. (1992) Dopamine agonists and pituitary tumor shrinkage, Endocr Rev 13, pp. 220–240.

Bigazzi M, Ronga R, Lancrangan I, Ferraro S, Branconi F, Buzzoni P, Martorana G, Scarselli GF, Del Pozo E. (1979) A pregnancy in an acromegalic woman during bromocriptine treatment: Effects on growth hormone and prolactin in the maternal, fetal and amniotic fluid compartments. J Clin Endocrinol Metab; 48: 9-12.

Biller BM, Luciano A, Crosignani P, Molitch M, Olive D, Rebar R, Sanfilippo J, Webster J, Zacur H. (1999) Guidelines for the diagnosis and treatment of hyperprolactinaemia, J Reprod Med, 44 pp. 1075–1084.

Biller BM, Molitch ME, Vance ML, Cannistraro KB, Davis KR, Simons JA, Schoenfelder JR, Klibanski A. (1996) Treatment of prolactin-secreting macroadenomas with the once-weekly dopamine agonist cabergoline, J Clin Endocrinol Metab 81, pp. 2338–2343.

Blackwell RE, Boots LR, Goldenberg RL, Younger JB. (1979) Assessment of pituitary function in patients with serum prolactin levels greater than 100 ng/ml. Fertil. Steril. 32, pp. 177–182.

Bole-Feysot C, Goffin V, Edery M, Binart N, Kelly PA. (1998) Prolactin (PRL) and its receptor: actions, signal transduction pathways and phenotypes observed in PRL receptor knockout mice, Endocr Rev 19:225.

Bracero N and Zacur HA. (2001) Polycystic ovary syndrome and hyperprolactinemia, Obstet Gynecol Clin North Am 28, pp. 77–84.

Bronstein MD, Musolino NR, Benabou S, Marino R Jr.(1989) Cerebrospinal fluid rhinorrhea occurring in long-term bromocriptine treatment for macroProlactinomas. Surg Neurol. 32(5):346-9.

Brooks DJ. (2000) Dopamine agonists: their role in the treatment of Parkinson's disease, J Neurol Neurosurg Psychiatry 68, pp. 685–689.

Brue T, Caruso E, Morange I, Hoffmann T, Evrin M, Gunz G, Benkirane M, Jaquet P. (1992) Immunoradiometric analysis of circulating human glycosylated and nonglycosylated prolactin forms: spontaneous and stimulated secretions, J Clin Endocrinol Metab 75:1338.

Cannavò S, Curtò L, Squadrito S, Almoto B, Vieni A, Trimarchi F. (1999) Cabergoline: a first-choice treatment in patients with previously untreated prolactin-secreting pituitary adenoma. J Endocrinol Invest; 22: 354-359.

Casanueva FF, Molitch ME, Schlechte JA, Abs R, Bonert V, Bronstein MD, Brue T, Cappabianca P, Colao A, Fahlbusch R, Fideleff H, Hadani M, Kelly P, Kleinberg D, Laws E, Marek J, Scanlon M, Sobrinho LG, Wass JA, Giustina A. (2006) Guidelines of the Pituitary Society for the diagnosis and management of prolactinomas, Clin Endocrinol (Oxf) 65, pp. 265–273.

Claxton AJ, Cramer J, Pierce C. (2001) A systematic review of the associations between dose regimens and medication compliance, Clin Ther 23, pp. 1296–1310.

Colao A, Annunziato L, Lombardi G. (1998) Treatment of prolactinomas. Ann med.30: 452-459.

Colao A, Di Sarno A, Cappabianca P, Di Somma C, Pivonello R, Lombardi G. (2003) Withdrawal of long-term cabergoline therapy for tumoural and nontumoural hyperprolactinemia, New Eng J Med 349:2023.

Colao A, Di sarno A, Landi ML, Scavuzzo F, Cappabianca P, Pivonello R, Volpe R, Di Salle F, Cirillo S, Annunziato L, Lombardi G. (2000) Macroprolactinoma shrinkage during cabergoline treatment is great in naïve patients than in patients pretreated with other dopamine agonists: a prospective study in 100 patients. J Clin Endocrinol Metab; 85: 2247-2252.

Conner P and Fried G. (1998) Hyperprolactinaemia; etiology, diagnosis and treatment alternatives. Acta Obstet Gynecol Scand. 77(3):249-62.

Cook CB, Nippoldt TB, Kletter GB, Kelch RP, Marshall JC. (1991) Naloxone increases the frequency of pulsatile luteinizing hormone secretion in women with hyperprolactinaemia, J Clin Endocrinol Metab 73:1099.

Corenblum B, Webster BR, Mortimer CB. (1975) Possible antitumour effect of CB 154 in 2 patients with large prolactin secreting pituitary adenomas. Clin. Res. 23, p. 614A.

Cuellar FG. (1980) Bromocriptine mesylate (Parlodel) in the management of amenorrhea/galactorrhea associated with hyperprolactinaemia. Obstet Gynecol; 55: 278.

Czeizel A, Kiss R, Racz K, Mohori K, Glaz E. (1989) Case-control cytogenetic study in offspring of mothers treated with bromocriptine during early pregnancy, Mutat Res 210, pp. 23–27.

Darwish AM, Emad Farah, Wafaa A. Gadallah, Ibraheem I Mohammad (2007) Superiority of newly developed vaginal suppositories over vaginal use of commercial bromocriptine tablets: a randomized controlled clinical trial. Reproductive Sciences 14(3);280-85.

Darwish AM, Ahmad M El-Sayed, Suasan A El-Harrasb (Late), Khaled A Khaled, Mohamad A Ismail (2008) Clinical Efficacy of Novel Unidirectional Buccoadhesive vs. Vaginoadhesive Bromocriptine mesylate Discs for Treating Pathologic Hyperprolactinemia. Fertil Steril. 90(5):1864-8.

Darwish AM, Ehsan Hafez, Ibraheem El-Gebali, Sahar B. Hassan, Mohammad E. Ali (2007) Rectal versus vaginal bromocriptine mesylate suppositories in hyperprolactinemic patients : an active comparator trial . MEFS Journal 12,2:25-29

Darwish AM, Hafez E, El-Gebaly I, Hassan SB. (2005) Evaluation of a novel vaginal bromocriptine mesylate formulation: A pilot study. Fertil Steril 83(4):1053-5.

Davis JR. (2004) Prolactin and reproductive medicine, Curr Opin Obstet Gynecol 16, pp. 331–337.

De Luis DA, Becerra A, Lahera M, Botella JI, Valero, Varela C. (2000) A randomized cross-over study comparing cabergoline and quinagolide in the treatment of hyperprolactinaemic patients. J Endocrinol Invest; 23: 428-434.

Del Pozo E, Del Re RB, Varga L, Friesen H. (1972) The inhibition of prolactin secretion in man by CB-154 (2-Br-alpha-ergocryptine). J Clin Endocrinol Metab. 35: 768-771.

Di Sarno A, Landi ML, Cappabianca P, Di Salle F, Rossi FW, Pivonello R, Di Somma C, Faggiano A, Lombardi G, Colao A. (2001) Resistance to cabergoline as compared with bromocriptine in hyperprolactinemia: prevalence, clinical definition, and therapeutic strategy, J Clin Endocrinol Metab 86, pp. 5256–5261.

Di Sarno A, Landi ML, Marzullo P, Di Somma C, Pivonello R, Cerbone G, Lombardi G, Colao A. (2000) The effect of quinagolide and cabergoline, two selective dopamine receptor type 2 agonists, in the treatment of prolactinomas, Clin Endocrinol (Oxford) 53, pp. 53–60.

Espinos JJ, Rodriguez-Espinosa J, Webb SM, Calaf-Alsina J. (1994) Long-acting repeatable bromocriptine in the treatment of patients with microprolactinoma intolerant or resistant to oral dopaminergics. Fertil Steril; 62: 926-931.

Essais O, Bouguerra R, Hamzaoui J, Marrakchi Z, Hadjri S, Chamakhi S, Zidi B, Ben Slama C. (2002) Efficacy and safety of bromocriptine in the treatment of macroprolactinomas, Ann Endocrinol (Paris) 63, pp. 524–531.

Factor SA. (1999) Dopamine agonists. Med Clin North Am. 83: 415-433.

Ferrari C, Barbieri C, Caldara R, Mucci M, Codecasa F, Paracchi A, Romano C, Boghen M, Dubini A. (1986) Long-lasting prolactin-lowering effect of cabergoline, a new dopamine agonist, in hyperprolactinaemic patients. J Clin Endocrinol Metab; 63: 941-945.

Ferrari CI, Abs R, Bevan JS, Brabant G, Ciccarelli E, Motta T, Mucci M, Muratori M, Musatti L, Verbessem G, Scanlon MF. (1997) Treatment of macroprolactinoma with cabergoline: a study of 85 patients, Clin Endocrinol (Oxford) 46, pp. 409–413.

Filopanti, AG Lania , A Spada (2010) Pharmacogenetics of D2 dopamine receptor gene in PRL-secreting pituitary adenomas. Expert Opin Drug Metab Toxicol. 6(1):43-53.

Franks S, Horrocks PM, Lynch SS, Butt WR, London DR. (1983) Effectiveness of pergolide mesylate in long term treatment of hyperprolactinaemia, Brit Med J (Clin Res Ed) 286 (1983), pp. 1177–1179.

Freda PU, Andreadis CI, Khandji AG, Khoury M, Bruce JN, Jacobs TP, Wardlaw SL. (2000) Long-term treatment of prolactin-secreting macroadenomas with pergolide. J Clin Endocrinol Metab; 85: 8-13.

Friedman E, Adams EF, Höög A, Gejman PV, Carson E, Larsson C, De Marco L, Werner S, Fahlbusch R, Nordenskjöld M. (1994) Normal structural dopamine type 2 receptor gene in prolactin secreting and other pituitary tumours. J. Clin. Endocrinol. Metab. 78, pp. 568–574.

Ginsburg J, Hardiman P, Thomas M (1992). Vaginal bromocriptine– clinical and biochemical effects. Gynecol Endocrinol 6:119 -26.

Giusti M, Porcella E, Carraro A, Cuttica M, Valenti S, Giordano G. (1994) A cross-over study with the two novel dopaminergic drugs cabergoline and quinagolide in hyperprolactinaemic patients. J Endocrinol Invest; 17: 51-57.

Glasser B, Nesher Y, Barziliai S. (1994) Long-term treatment of bromocriptine-intolerant prolactinoma patients with CV205-502. J Reprod Med; 39: 449-454.

Glazener CM, Kelly NJ, Hull MG (1987). PRL measurement in the investigation of infertility in women with a normal menstrual cycle. Br J Obstet Gynaecol. 94(6):535-8.

Gregg C, Shikar V, Larsen P, Mak G, Chojnacki A, Yong VW, Weiss S. (2007) White matter plasticity and enhanced remyelination in the maternal CNS. Journal of Neuroscience 27(8): 1812-1823.

Hall WA, Luciano MG, Doppman JL, Patronas NJ, Oldfield EH. (1994) Pituitary magnetic resonance imaging in normal human volunteers: Occult adenomas in general populations. Ann Internal Med; 120:817.

Hattori N and Inagaki C. (1997) Anti-prolactin (PRL) autoantibodies cause asymptomatic hyperprolactinaemia: bioassay and clearance studies of PRL-immunoglobulin G complex, J Clin Endocrinol Metab 82:3107.

Hattori N, Ishihara T, Ikekubo K, Moridera K, Hino M, Kurahachi H. (1992) Autoantibody to human prolactin in patients with idiopathic hyperprolactinaemia, J Clin Endocrinol Metab 75:1226.

Hawkins T. (2004) Impact of once- and twice-daily dosing regimens on adherence and overall safety, AIDS Reader 14, pp. 320–322 324, 329–31, 334–6.

Hewage UC, Colman PG, Kaye A (2000). Cerebrospinal fluid (CSF) rhinorrhoea occurring six days after commencement of bromocriptine for invasive macro Prolactinoma. Aust N Z J Med. 30(3):399-400.

Ho KY and Thorner MO. (1988) Therapeutic applications of bromocriptine in endocrine and neurological diseases, Drugs 36, pp. 67–82.

Hofmann C, Penner U, Dorow R, Pertz HH, Jähnichen S, Horowski R, Latté KP, Palla D, Schurad B (2006) Lisuride, a dopamine receptor agonist with 5-HT2B receptor antagonist properties: absence of cardiac valvulopathy adverse drug reaction reports supports the concept of a crucial role for 5-HT2B receptor agonism in cardiac valvular fibrosis. Clin Neuropharmacol. 29(2):80-6.

Homburg R, West C, Brownell J, Jacobs HS. (1990) A double-blind study comparing a new non-ergot, long-acting dopamine agonist, CV 205–502, with bromocriptine in women with hyperprolactinaemia, Clin Endocrinol (Oxford) 32 , pp. 565–571.

Hou SH, Grossman S, Molitch ME. (1985) Hyperprolactinaemia in patient with renal insufficiency and chronic renal failure requiring haemodialysis or chronic ambulatory peritoneal dialysis. Am. J. Kidney Dis. 6, pp. 245–249.

Hutchinson SM and Zacur HA. (1997) Hyperprolactinemia after laparoscopic ovarian drilling: an unknown phenomenon. Treatment of infertility with dopamine agonists, In: Seible Med. Infertility, 2nd ed. Stamford, CT: Appleton & Lange: 557-569.

Ilkko E, Tikkakoski T, Salmela P, Pyhtinen J, Kurunlahti M. (2002) MR imaging of pituitary adenomas treated with the prolactin inhibitor quinagolide. Acta Radiol; 43: 125-129.

Jackson RD, Wortsman J, Malarkey WB. (1985) Characterization of a large molecular weight prolactin in women with idiopathic hyperprolactinaemia and normal menses, J Clin Endocrinol Metab 61:258.

Jeffcoate WJ, Pound N, Sturrock NDC, Lambourne J. (1996) Long-term follow-up of patients with hyperprolactinaemia. Clin. Endocrinol. 45, pp. 299–303.

Jose PA, Eisner GM, Felder RA. (1998) Renal dopamine receptors in health and hypertension, Pharmacol Ther 80, pp. 149–182.

Karagianis J and Baksh A. (2003) High dose olanzapine and prolactin levels, J Clin Psychiatry 64, pp. 1192–1194.

Karavitaki N, Thanabalasingham G, Shore HC, Trifanescu R, Ansorge O, Meston N, Turner HE, Wass JA. (2006) Do the limits of serum prolactin in disconnection hyperprolactinaemia need re-definition? A study of 226 patients with histologically verified non-functioning pituitary macroadenoma, Clin Endocrinol (Oxf) 65, pp. 524–529.

Katz E, Schran HF, Adashi EY. (1989) Successful treatment of a prolactin producing macroadenoma with intravaginal bromocriptine mesylate: a novel approach to intolerance of oral therapy. Obstet. Gynecol. 73, pp. 517–520.

Kaye TB. (1996) Hyperprolactinaemia. Causes, consequences, and treatment options. Postgrad Med. May; 99(5):265-8.

Kostrzak A, Warenik-Szymankiewicz A, Meczekalski B (2009). The role of serum PRL bioactivity evaluation in hyperprolactinemic women with different menstrual disorders. Gynecol Endocrinol. 25(12):799-806.

Lamberts SW and Quik RF. (1991) A comparison of the efficacy and safety of pergolide and bromocriptine in the treatment of hyperprolactinaemia. J Clin Endocrinol Metab; 72: 635-641.

Lappohn RE, van de Wiel HBM, Brownell J. (1992) The effect of two dopaminergic drugs on menstrual function and psychological state in hyperprolactinaemia, Fertil Steril 58:321.

Levey AI, Hersch SM, Rye DB, Sunahara RK, Niznik HB, Kitt CA, Price DL, Maggio R, Brann MR, Ciliax BJ. (1993) Localization of D1 and D2 dopamine receptors in brain with subtype-specific antibodies, Proc Natl Acad Sci USA 90, pp. 8861–8865.

Luque EH, Munoz de Toro M, Smith PF, Neill JD. (1986) Subpopulations of lactotropes detected with the reverse hemolytic plaque assay show differential responsiveness to dopamine. Endocrinology; 118: 2120-2124.

Mah PM and Webster J. (2002) Hyperprolactinaemia: etiology, diagnosis, and management, Seminars Reprod Med 20, pp. 365–374.

Mannelli M, Lazzeri C, Ianni L, La Villa G, Pupilli C, Bellini F, Serio M, Franchi F. (1997) Dopamine and sympathoadrenal activity in man, Clin Exp Hypertens 19, pp. 163–179.

Matera C, Freda PU, Ferin M, Wardlaw SL. (1995) Effect of chronic opioid antagonism on the hypothalamic-pituitary-ovarian axis in hyperprolactinaemic women, J Clin Endocrinol Metab 80:540.

Melmed S. (1997) The structure and function of pituitary dopamine receptors, Endocrinologist 7:385.

Melmed S. Disorders of the anterior pituitary and hypothalamus. In: (Braunwald, et al; 2001).

Merola B, Colao A, Caruso E, Sarnacchiaro F, Briganti F, Lancranjan I, et al. (1989). Oral and injectable long-acting bromocriptine preparations in mesylate: a novel approach to intolerance of oral therapy. Obstet Gynecol 73:517–20.

Milewicz A. (1984) Prolactin levels in the polycystic ovary syndrome, J Reprod Med 29, pp. 193–196.

Molitch ME. (2001) Disorders of prolactin secretion, Endocrinol Metab Clin North Am 30, pp. 585–610.

Morange I, Barlier A, Pellegrini I, Brue T, Enjalbert A, Jaquet P. (1996) Prolactinomas resistant to bromocriptine: long-term efficacy of quinagolide and outcome of pregnancy, Eur J Endocrinol 135, pp. 413–420.

Mori H, Mori S, Saitoh Y, Arita N, Aono T, Uozumi T, Mogami H, Matsumoto K. (1985) Effects of bromocriptine on prolactin secreting pituitary adenomas. Cancer 56, pp. 230–238.

Moriondo P, Travaglini P, Nissim M, Conti A, Faglia G. (1985) Bromocriptine treatment of microprolactinomas: evidence of stable prolactin decrease after drug withdrawal, J Clin Endocrinol Metab 60, pp. 764–772.

Motta T, de Vincentiis S, Marchini M, Colombo N, D'Alberton A. (1996) Vaginal cabergoline in the treatment of hyperprolactinaemic patients intolerant to oral dopaminergics, Fertil Steril 65:440.

Moyle G. (2003) Once-daily therapy: less is more, Int J STD AIDS 14 (Suppl 1), pp. 1–5.

Netea-Maier RT, van Lindert EJ, Timmers H, Schakenraad EL, Grotenhuis JA, Hermus AR. Cerebrospinal fluid leakage as complication of treatment with cabergoline for macroProlactinomas. J Endocrinol Invest. 2006 Dec;29(11):1001-5.

Nordmann R, Fluckiger EW, Petcher TJ, Brownell J. (1988) Endocrine actions of the potent dopamine D-2 agonist CV205-502 and related octahydrobenzo- (g) -quinolines. Drugs of the future; 13: 951-959.

Nunes V, El Dib R, Boguszewski C, Nogueira C (2011). Cabergoline versus bromocriptine in the treatment of HP: a systematic review of randomized controlled trials and meta-analysis Pituitary . Volume: 14, Issue: 3, Pages: 259-265.

Orrego JJ, Chandler WF, Barkan AL. (2000) Pergolide as primary therapy for macroprolactinomas. Pituitary; 3: 251-256.

Parsanezhad ME, Alborzi S, Zolghadri J, Parsa-Nezhad M, Keshavarzi G, Omrani GR, Schmidt EH (2005). Hyperprolactinemia after laparoscopic ovarian drilling: an unknown phenomenon. Reprod Biol Endocrinol. 7;3:31.

Pellegrini I, Rasolonjanahary R, Gunz G, Bertrand P, Delivet S, Jedynak CP, Kordon C, Peillon F, Jaquet P, Enjalbert A. (1989) Resistance to bromocriptine in prolactinomas, J Clin Endocrinol Metab 69, pp. 500–509.

Peter SA, Autz A, Jean-Simon ML. (1993) Bromocriptine-induced schizophrenia, J Natl Med Assoc 85, pp. 700–701.

Pontikides N, Krassas GE, Nikopoulou E, Kaltsas T. (2000) Cabergoline as a first-line treatment in newly diagnosed macroprolactinomas. Pituitary; 2: 277-281.

Porcile A, Gallardo E, Venegas E. (1990) Normoprolactinaemic anovulation nonresponsive to clomiphin citrate: Ovulation induction with bromocriptine. Fertil Steril; 53: 50.

Quinn AM, Rubinas TC, Garbincius CJ, Holmes EW (2006). Determination of ultrafilterable PRL: elimination of macroprolactin interference with a monomeric PRL-selective sample pretreatment. Arch Pathol Lab Med. 130(12):1807-12.

Rains CP, Bryson HM, Fitton A. (1995) Cabergoline, A review of its pharmacological properties and therapeutic potential in the treatment of hyperprolactinaemia and inhibition of lactation, Drugs 49, pp. 255–279.

Rasmussen C, Brownell J, Bergh T. (1991) Clinical response and prolactin concentration in hyperprolactinaemic women during and after treatment for 24 months with the new dopamine agonist, CV 205-502. Acta Endocrinol (Copenh); 125: 170-176.

Rennert J and Doerfler A. (2007) Imaging of sellar and parasellar lesions, Clin Neurol Neurosurg 109, pp. 111–124.

Ricci G, Giolo E, Nucera G. (2001) Pregnancy in hyperprolactinaemic infertile women treated with vaginal bromocriptine: report of two cases and review of the literature. Gynecol Obstet Invest; 51: 266-270.

Rizzo JA and Simons WR. (1997) Variations in compliance among hypertensive patients by drug class: implications for health care costs, Clin Ther 19, pp. 1446–1457 discussion 1424–1445.

Robert E, Musatti L, Piscitelli G, Ferrari CI. (1996) Pregnancy outcome after treatment with the ergot derivative, cabergoline. Reprod Toxicol; 10: 333-337.

Schilling JC, Adams WS, Palluk R. (1992) Neuroendocrine side effects profile of pramipexole, a new dopamine receptor agonist, in humans. Clin Pharmacol Ther; 51: 541-548.

Schlechte J, Sherman B, Halmi N, Van Gilder J, Chapler FK, Dolan K, Granner D, Duello T, Harris C. (1980) Prolactin-secreting pituitary tumours, Endocr Rev 1:295.

Schofl C, Schofl-Siegert B, Karstens JH, Bremer M, Lenarz T, Cuarezma JS, Samii M, von zur Muhlen A, Brabant G. (2002) Falsely low serum prolactin in two cases of invasive macroprolactinoma, Pituitary 5:261.

Schoors DF, Vauquelin GP, De Vos H, Smets G, Velkeniers B, Vanhaelst L, Dupont AG. (1991) Identification of a D1 dopamine receptor not linked to adenylate cyclase, on lactotroph cells, Brit J Pharmacol 103, pp. 1928–1934.

Schultz PN, Ginsberg L, McCutcheon IE, Samaan N, Leavens M, Gagel RF. (2000) Quinagolide in the management of prolactinoma, Pituitary 3, pp. 239–249.

Shelesnyak MC. (1958) Maintenance of gestation in ergotoxine treated pregnant rats by exogenous prolactin. Actn Endocrinol (Kbh). 27: 99-109.

Smith TP, Suliman AM, Fahie-Wilson MN, McKenna TJ. (2002) Gross variability in the detection of prolactin in sera containing big big prolactin (macroprolactin) by commercial immunoassays, J Clin Endocrinol Metab 87:5410.

Snyder JM and Dekowski SA. (1992) The role of prolactin in fetal lung maturation, Seminars Reprod Endocrinol 10:287.

Soule SG and Jacob HS. (1995) Prolactinoma: Present day management. Br J Obstet Gynecol; 102: 178-181.

Speroff L, Levin RM, Haning RV, Jr., Kase NG. (1979) A practical approach for the evaluation of women with abnormal polytomography or elevated prolactin levels, Am J Obstet Gynecol 135:896.

Stein AL, Levenick MN, Kletzky OA. (1989) Computed tomography versus magnetic resonance imaging for the evaluation of suspected pituitary adenomas, Obstet Gynecol 73:996.

Strebel PM, Zacur HA, Gold EB. (1986) Headache, hyperprolactinemia, and prolactinomas, Obstet Gynecol 68:195.

Tamura T, Satoh T, Minakami H, Tamada T. (1989) Effects of hydergeine in hyperprolactinaemia. J Clin Endocrinol Metab; 69: 470-474.

Teasdale E, Teasdale G, Mohsen F, MacPherson P. (1986) High-resolution computed tomography in pituitary microadenoma: is seeing believing?, Clin Radiol 37:227.

Testa G, Vegetti W, Motta T, Alagna F, Bianchedi D, Carlucci C, Bianchi M, Parazzini F, Crosignani PG. (1998) Two-year treatment with oral contraceptives in hyperprolactinaemic patients, Contraception 58:69-73.

Touraine P, Plu-Bureau G, Beji C, Mauvais-Jarvis P, Kuttenn F. (2001) Long-term follow-up of 246 hyperprolactinaemic patients, Acta Obstet Gynecol Scand 80, pp. 162–168.

Turkalj I, Braun P, Krupp P. (1982) Surveillance of bromocriptine in pregnancy. JAMA; 247: 1589-1591.

Valdemarsson S. (2004) Macroprolactinaemia. Risk of misdiagnosis and mismanagement in hyperprolactinaemia. Lakartidningen; 101(6): 458-465.

Vallar L, Vicentini LM, Meldolesi J. (1988) Inhibition of inositol phosphate production is a late, Ca2+-dependent effect of D2 dopaminergic receptor activation in rat lactotroph cells, J Biol Chem 263, pp. 10127–10134.

Vallette-Kasic S, Morange-Ramos I, Selim A, Gunz G, Morange S, Enjalbert A, Martin P-M, Jaquet P, Brue T. (2002) Macroprolactinaemia revisited: a study on 106 patients, J Clin Endocrinol Metab 87:581-588.

Van der Lely AJ, Brownell J, Lamberts SW. (1991) The efficacy and tolerability of CV205-502 (a nonergot dopaminergic drug) in macroprolactinoma patients and in prolactinoma patients intolerant to bromocriptine. J Clin Endocrinol Metab; 72: 1136-1141.

Van't Verlaat JW and Croughs RJ. (1991) Withdrawal of bromocriptine after long-term therapy for macroprolactinomas; effect on plasma prolactin and tumour size, Clin Endocrinol (Oxford) 34, pp. 175–178.

Vance ML, Evans WS, Thorner MO. (1984) Drugs 5 years later. Bromocriptine, Ann Intern Med 100, pp. 78–91.

Verhelst J, Abs R, Maiter D, van den Bruel A, Vandeweghe M, Velkeniers B, Mockel J, Lamberigts G, Petrossians P, Coremans P, Mahler C, Stevenaert A, Verlooy J, Raftopoulos C, Beckers A. (1999) Cabergoline in the treatment of hyperprolactinaemia: a study of 455 patients. J Clin Endocrinol Metab; 84: 2518-2522.

Webster J. (1999) Clinical management of prolactinomas, Baillieres Best Pract Res Clin Endocrinol Metab 13, pp. 395–408.

Weil C. (1986) The safety of bromocriptine in hyperprolactinaemic female infertility: a literature review. Curr Med Res Opin; 10: 172-195.

Weingrill CO, Mussio W, Moraes CRY, Portes E, Castro RC, Lengyel AM. (1992) Long-acting oral bromocriptine (Parlodel SRO) in the treatment of hyperprolactinaemia. Fertil Steril.; 57: 331-335.

Whitaker MD, Klee GG, Kas KP. (1983) Demonstration of biological activity of prolactin molecular weight variants in human sera, J. Clin. Endocrinol. Metab. 58, p. 826.

Wilson JD. (1998) Endocrine disorders of the breast. In: Braunwald E, Isselbacher KJ, Wilson J, et al, eds. Harrison's Principles of Internal Medicine. 14th ed. New York, NY: McGraw-Hill; 2116-2117.

Yuen YP, Lai JP, Au KM, Chan AY, Mak TW. (2003) Macroprolactin-a cause of pseudohyperprolactinaemia, Hong Kong Med J 9, pp. 119–121.

Zacur HA, Foster GV, Tyson JE. (1976) Multifactorial regulation of prolactin secretion. Lancet. 1: 410-413.

Zeilmaker GH and Carslen RA. (1962) Experimental studies on the effect of ergocornine methane sulfonate on the lutealtrophic function of the rat pituitary gland. Acta Endocrinol (Kbh).41: 321-335.

2

Ovarian Follicular Atresia

David H. Townson[1,*] and Catherine M.H. Combelles[2]
[1]*University of New Hampshire, Department of Molecular, Cellular and Biomedical Sciences, Durham NH,*
[2]*Middlebury College, Department of Biology, Middlebury VT, USA*

1. Introduction

Throughout ovarian development and function in mammals, a highly orchestrated, periodic process known as follicular atresia occurs that destroys and eliminates follicles and oocytes from the ovary. Follicular atresia is pervasive. In humans, it is estimated to account for 99.9% of the loss of oocytes from development of the fetal ovary until reproductive senescence (Baker, 1963; Faddy et al., 1992). Overall, the process of follicular atresia eliminates all but 300-400 oocytes, some of which become available for selection, ovulation and potential fertilization. Similar phenomena of loss are observed in other mammals. The rationale for such extensive elimination of oocytes during fetal and adult life is unknown. However, in the case of larger, more mature follicles (i.e., antral follicles), the importance of follicular atresia is attributed to a finite lifespan of the oocyte. Hence, in the adult female, atresia ensures that only the healthiest follicles, containing oocytes of optimal quality for fertilization, remain available throughout the reproductive period. In this chapter, we provide a broad overview of the physiological process of follicular atresia, giving emphasis to the cellular and molecular mechanisms that influence the process in two monovulatory species, the cow and human female.

2. Follicular development and classification of follicles

Prior to the onset of follicular atresia, the ovary contains an abundance of non-dividing, primordial follicles, which contain the reserve of germ cells available for fertilization throughout the reproductive life of the adult. Primordial follicles consist of an immature oocyte surrounded by a single layer of granulosa cells. In many mammals the number of primordial follicles is established at the time of birth, whereas in the human female and in many domesticated livestock, including the cow, this number is determined during fetal development. In either scenario the transition from non-dividing/non-growing primordial follicles to growing follicles is a critical part of follicular development or "folliculogenesis". It is a process that begins gradually, almost imperceptibly after the formation of primordial follicles, and then continues throughout the reproductive life of the animal (Fortune et al., 1998; Oktem & Urman, 2010). However, the factors influencing the formation of primordial

* Corresponding Author

follicles and the mechanism(s) responsible for their activation are largely unknown and beyond the scope of this review. A recent article by Aerts and Bols (Aerts & Bols, 2010) provides insight about these topics as they pertain to the cow, which may be informative for the reader. Here, the discussion will focus on literature concerning folliculogenesis and follicular atresia beyond that of the primordial follicle. In addition, studies emphasizing bovine (cow) and human ovarian function will be highlighted because both species are principally monovulatory (i.e., release one oocyte for fertilization per estrous/menstrual cycle), and both entail similar follicular dynamics in which development, selection and dominance of a single follicle occurs from, and at the expense of, a cohort of growing follicles.

A general classification of follicles in the adult ovary consists of the following four categories: 1) Primordial follicles, 2) Primary follicles, 3) Secondary follicles, and 4) Tertiary follicles (General characteristics are summarized in Table 1). Primordial follicles consist of a single layer of granulosa cells (< 10 cells total) surrounding an immature oocyte (~30um) with no zona pellucida. Overall follicle diameter is <40 um. Primary follicles are comprised of one to two layers of cuboidal granulosa cells (10-40 cells) surrounding an immature, spherical oocyte (25-45 um). Sparse patches of zona pellucida are evident around the oocyte. Ultrastructurally, the mitochondria of the oocyte are "round" and located in the deep cortical region. Golgi complexes are also located in the deep cortical region with junctional adherins detectable between the oocyte and the surrounding granulosa cells. The oocyte also contains extensive rough and smooth endoplasmic reticulum, but no cortical granules or microtubules (Gougeon & Chainy, 1987; Fair et al., 1997; Kacinskis et al., 2005; Westergaard et al., 2007). Secondary follicles have two to six layers of cuboidal granulosa cells (40-250 cells) surrounding a maturing oocyte (35-70um). Small amounts of zona pellucida surround the oocyte in half the follicles. Ultrastructural features include erect microvilli of the oocyte peneterating the zona pellucida, gap junctions between the oocyte and surrounding granulosa cells, "elongated" mitochondria in the deep cortical region, extensive rough and smooth endoplasmic reticulum, clusters of cortical granules in a few oocytes, but again, no microtubules (Gougeon & Chainy, 1987; Fair et al., 1997; Kacinskis et al., 2005). Tertiary follicles have greater than six layers of granulosa cells (>250 cells), which contain a mature oocyte (100-150um) and a fully-formed zona pellucida surrounded by specialized granulosa cells called the cumulus oophorus. The oocyte of these follicles contain erect microvilli which traverse the zona pellucida, gap and adherens junctions, abundant round and elongated mitochondria, extensive rough and smooth endoplasmic reticulum, numerous lipid droplets and vesicles, increased numbers of Golgi, clusters of cortical granules in all oocytes, and vast arrays of microtubules (Fair *et al.*, 1997). Tertiary follicles are most notably distinguished by the presence of a fluid-filled antrum which, in the case of the bovine, results in follicles of 0.5 to 25mm in diameter. In addition to the above general characteristics and classification of follicles, specialized cells derived from the ovarian stroma, called theca cells, surround the basal lamina of primary follicles (Hirshfield, 1991), but later form distinct layers of theca interna and externa as the follicles transition from secondary to tertiary status. Throughout the reproductive life of the female, any and all of the above types of follicles are evident histologically within the ovary. For further review about the classifications and descriptions of ovarian follicles, the reader is referred to the following authors (Mossman & Duke, 1973; Gougeon & Chainy, 1987; Fair et al., 1997; Kacinskis et al., 2005; Westergaard et al., 2007).

Follicle Category	Granulosa Layer	Oocyte Characteristics	Other Characteristics
Primordial Follicles	Single layer, cuboidal cells (<10 cells)	Immature oocyte (~30 microns; no zona pellucida)	Follicle diameter <40 microns
Primary Follicles	One to two layers, cuboidal cells (10-40 cells)	Immature, spherical oocyte (25-45 microns; sparse zona pellucida)	"Round" mitochondria, golgi complexes in deep cortical region of oocyte
Secondary Follicles	Two to six layers, cuboidal cells (40-250 cells)	Maturing oocyte (35-70 microns; small amounts of zona pellucida)	Erect microvilli of oocyte penetrate the zona pellucida, "Elongated" mitochondria, extensive smooth and rough endoplasmic reticulum
Tertiary Follicles	More than six layers, squamous cells (>250 cells)	Mature oocyte (100-150 microns; fully formed zona pellucida)	Presence of cumulus oophorus, extensive organelle development within the oocyte, antrum formation

Table 1. General classification and characteristics of follicles of the adult ovary. Morphometric and ultrastructural characteristics of follicles are further described by Gougeon & Chainy, 1987; Fair et al., 1997; Kacinskis et al., 2005; and Westergaard et al., 2007.

3. Characteristics of growth of antral follicles

In the cow, growth of follicles is an ongoing process, beginning with the growth of primordial follicles around day 90 of fetal gestation (Fortune, 2003; Fortune et al., 2010, 2011). These follicles develop into primary, secondary, and early tertiary (preantral) follicles in the absence of gonadotropins, with late tertiary, antral follicles beginning to emerge near day 210 of gestation (Yang & Fortune, 2008). Thereafter, especially following puberty, pituitary gonadotropins and locally-secreted ovarian modulators prompt the growth of cohorts of tertiary follicles within both ovaries, and facilitate the selection of a single follicle suitable for ovulation and conception. Tertiary follicles develop into mature, preovulatory-size follicles within 42 days, encompassing approximately the period of two estrous cycles in cows. Among the many hormones that stimulate the growth and development of these follicles, follicle-stimulating hormone (FSH) is recognized as a major influence.

Systemic, pulsatile secretion of FSH triggers the synchronous development of a cohort of tertiary follicles in the ovary of the cow during the estrous cycle, which is often referred to as a "follicular wave". The emergence of these waves coincides temporally with a surge of FSH secretion (Adams *et al.*, 1992), during which one or two dominant follicles and several subordinate follicles develop (Savio et al., 1988; Sirois & Fortune, 1988; Knopf et al., 1989). Most estrous cycles of the cow consist of two or three waves of follicular growth preceding ovulation. A similar pattern of follicular growth during the menstrual cycle occurs in women (Baerwald *et al.*, 2003). Interestingly, granulosa cells of follicles express FSH receptors relatively early in follicular development, particularly in primary follicles (Oktay et al., 1997; Bao & Garverick, 1998; Findlay & Drummond, 1999; Webb et al., 1999).

Conceptually it is reasonable to suggest pulsatile FSH secretion might also influence the growth of primary and secondary follicles, but this possibility has not yet been adequately explored. Regardless, we know that during a follicular wave a cohort of tertiary follicles emerges as a result of FSH stimulation. One follicle is selected and becomes dominant; whereas the remaining follicles of the cohort become subordinates (Ginther *et al.*, 1997). Dominant follicles secrete hormones that play a prominent role in their continued growth while simultaneously limiting the growth and possibly triggering the regression of the subordinate follicles of the cohort. Inhibins, for instance, are secreted by dominant follicles, which then act systemically to diminish FSH secretion (Armstrong & Webb, 1997; Webb et al., 1999; Knight & Glister, 2006). Dominant follicles also maintain high levels of estradiol secretion, which further reduces FSH secretion and compromises the growth needs of the subordinate follicles (Ginther *et al.*, 2000). Insulin-like growth factor-1 (IGF-1), its binding proteins, and other growth factors are additional influences within the microenvironment of the ovary that impact the growth and dominance of follicles (Armstrong & Webb, 1997; Webb et al., 1999; Armstrong et al., 2000). Elevated concentrations of free insulin-like growth factor-1 (IGF-1) within the dominant follicle, for instance, support its continued development as the availability of FSH declines (Beg & Ginther, 2006). Concomitantly, dominant follicles acquire additional luteinizing hormone (LH) receptors to respond to increased LH availability and the preovulatory LH surge (Beg & Ginther, 2006). Although subordinate follicles also possess these developmental capabilities, they evidently lack sufficient time during the follicular wave to attain them and, hence, are destined to undergo regression in a process known as "follicular atresia".

4. Overview of follicular atresia

Based upon the etiomology of the word (from Greek: a= not, tresia=perforated), follicular atresia strictly refers to the failure of a follicle to rupture or ovulate. More broadly, follicular atresia encompasses the fate or demise of all follicles except those destined for ovulation. While most studies focus on follicular atresia in the adult ovary, the process also predominates in the fetal ovary and after birth. Before the time of follicle formation, and upon establishment within the developing ovary, the primordial germ cells become oogonia; while oogonia continue to proliferate, they are also subject to large-scale apoptotic demise. Around mid-gestation (about 20 weeks of fetal development in human), oogonia undergo transformation into oocytes that enter meiosis, but are later arrested at the dictyate stage. This is also the period when oocytes become surrounded by granulosa cells to form primordial follicles. In the human female fetus, the peak number of oocytes is reached at mid-gestation (~ 7 million cells), but during the last half of gestation at least two-thirds of these are lost, leaving a reserve of 1 to 2 million oocytes at birth. This massive loss of germ cells (named oocyte attrition) results from apoptosis of these cells at all developmental stages (Baker, 1963; Forabosco et al., 1991). Oocyte attrition also occurs prenatally before follicle formation. Of note is the observation in the bovine that any oocyte that fails to become part of a primordial follicle will be lost (Ohno & Smith, 1964). The loss of germ cells does not end at the time of birth; in the human female, there is an additional 75% loss of oocytes through puberty (with about 400,000 remaining within follicles) (Baker, 1963; Peters et al., 1978; Himelstein-Braw et al., 1976). In contrast to the prenatal situation, post-natal depletion of oocytes occurs by follicle atresia. Follicular development is characteristically dynamic throughout childhood, with the size of the follicle reserve at puberty being a reflection of the dynamic outcomes of follicular quiescence, growth, or atresia (Tingen et al., 2009). Throughout reproductive life, about 400 follicles will attain ovulation with an estimated 250,000 follicles lost by atresia at a rate of about 1000 follicles per month. However, the rate of follicular atresia is accelerated in the years preceding menopause (Faddy et al., 1992).

Follicular atresia affects all stages of follicular development, but the proportion of follicles that become atretic is enhanced by increased follicle size. In natural cycles, small antral follicles are particularly prone to atresia (Gosden & Spears, 1997; Hirshfield, 1991; Kaipia & Hsueh, 1997). With no new oocytes or follicles forming after birth, the subject of follicular loss is particularly poignant. The adult female mammal has only a finite number of follicles and there is a very high rate of follicular atresia. This suggests follicular atresia is under tight control to ensure oocytes remain available for ovulation throughout the reproductive life of the female. The regulation of follicular atresia is a topic presented below.

5. Antral versus basal follicular atresia in the cow

Histological descriptions of follicular atresia in the bovine ovary date back nearly 50 years. Among these, two studies in particular established classifications of atresia which differed (Rajakoski, 1960; Marion et al., 1968), and since may have contributed to the misinterpretation of findings by authors of more recent investigations. Irving-Rodgers and coworkers (Irving-Rodgers *et al.*, 2001) re-visited this subject and provided evidence for two basic morphological forms of atresia in cattle: 1) Antral atresia, and 2) Basal atresia. The general histological features of these two forms atresia are summarized below. However, more importantly, Irving-Rodgers and co-workers (Irving-Rodgers *et al.*, 2001) also suggested that more recent studies in which the previous classifications had been implemented to correlate with biochemical or physiological parameters of follicle status should be re-evaluated.

Antral atresia is characterized by the initial elimination of granulosa cells proximal to the antrum. Numerous pyknotic nuclei are evident in these antral layers of the membrana granulosa, and sometimes within the antrum itself. Remnants of mitochondrial and plasma membranes are also seen associated with the pyknotic nuclei (Irving-Rodgers *et al.*, 2001). The basal granulosa cells (i.e., those aligning the basal lamina), conversely, remain intact and possess many ultrastructural characteristics of healthy cells (e.g. moderate numbers of mitochondria, lipid droplets, and moderate amounts of endoplasmic reticulum)(Irving-Rodgers *et al.*, 2001). Antral atresia is viewed as the classic and most widely-observed form of follicular atresia because it occurs at all stages of follicle development in most species, and it is universally seen in large follicles (> 5 mm in diameter), including the dominant follicle, of monovulatory species (Irving-Rodgers *et al.*, 2001).

Basal atresia entails the destruction of the most basal layer of the follicle, whereas the most antral layers remain intact and healthy (Irving-Rodgers *et al.*, 2001). The basal lamina is often penetrated by macrophages and invading capillaries, and the theca layer of the follicle has additional deposition of collagen. The middle layers of the membrana granulosa exhibit a progression of cellular morphology and ultrastructure from the fragmented, pyknotic cells typical of the basal layers to the healthy, intact cells found in the antral layers. In the cow/heifer, this form of atresia occurs only in small follicles (< 5 mm in diameter)(Irving-Rodgers *et al.*, 2001). Whether or not this form atresia is unique to the bovine is uncertain because, to date, there have been no other reports of its existence in other species.

6. Apoptosis as a mechanism of follicular atresia

Apoptosis is recognized as a hallmark and contributing factor of atresia of antral follicles (Tilly et al., 1991; Tilly, 1996; Chun & Hsueh, 1998; Johnson, 2003; Matsuda-Minehata et al., 2006; Inoue et al., 2011). It is a cell-specific mechanism of discrete elimination of cells during follicular atresia that ensures regression of the follicle without inciting an overt inflammatory response. During atresia the cells of the follicle undergoing apoptosis are generally scattered throughout the parenchyma, and may or may not include the oocyte (Kim et al., 1998; D'Haeseleer et al., 2006; Peluffo et al., 2007). Initiating mechanisms of apoptosis include extrinsic factors, such as the cytokines, and intrinsic factors including oxidative stress, irradiation, and the activation of tumor suppressor genes.

Cytokines are among the extrinsic factors of apoptosis because their effects are initiated extracellularly through receptor-mediated mechanisms. Members of the tumor necrosis factor (TNF) superfamily are among the most widely-recognized cytokines triggering apoptotic events in follicles. They include TNF (Basini et al., 2002; Sasson et al., 2002), Fas ligand (Porter *et al.*, 2000), and TNF-related apoptosis-inducing ligand (TRAIL)(Johnson et al., 2007; Jaaskelainen et al., 2009). Additional extrinsic factors that influence apoptosis of granulosa cells include interferon-gamma (Quirk et al., 2000; Vickers et al., 2000) and several types of growth factors (Quirk *et al.*, 2000). Intrinsic factors of apoptosis are those that are generally provoked by aspects of stress. For instance, nutrient deprivation, oxidative damage, and genetic impairment are all examples of cellular/molecular stress that can lead to the upregulation of intrinsic mechanisms of apoptosis.

Aspects of follicular growth, selection, and atresia are considered highly-orchestrated processes in which the ovarian microenvironment and the interplay between pro-apoptotic and anti-apoptotic molecules have a significant role. A fairly comprehensive review of many of these molecules, their actions, with accompanying references, has been described previously (Hussein, 2005). The complexity of the signaling pathways these molecules utilize, however, is not well understood, and the discovery of novel molecules and mechanisms which influence granulosa cell survival continues (Hennebold, 2010). For instance, the recent finding of a microRNA (*Mir21*), which blocks apoptosis of murine granulosa cells (Carletti *et al.*, 2010), indicates there may be a vast array of other molecular mechanisms controlling granulosa cell fate, and hence follicular fate, which have yet to be investigated.

Members of the tumor necrosis superfamily are perhaps among the most readily identified pro-apoptotic molecules associated with granulosa cell death and follicular atresia. In the human, bovine, and other species, Fas ligand and the Fas-mediated pathway of apoptosis are considered prominent mechanisms of granulosa cell death during follicular atresia (Quirk et al., 1995; Hakuno et al., 1996; Kondo et al., 1996; Vickers et al., 2000). The targeted, cell-specific nature of granulosa cell death without any accompanying inflammatory response or collateral damage to adjacent cells is a unique feature of the Fas ligand-Fas system, consistent with its renowned role(s) in immune response, the establishment of immune tolerance, and the activation-induced cell death of lymphocytes. The cytokines TNF, TRAIL, and their corresponding receptors are additional factors, similar to Fas ligand and Fas, that potentially influence cell fate and follicle status in certain species (Prange-Kiel et al., 2001; Xiao et al., 2002; Inoue et al., 2003). In general, cytokine binding and reception triggers the intracellular activation of initiator and effector caspases (Boone & Tsang, 1998; Johnson & Bridgham, 2002; Valdez et al., 2005; Hurst et al., 2006). Initiatior caspases include caspase-6, 8, 9 and 10, while effector caspases include caspase-2, 3, 6, 7 and 14 (McCarthy & Bennett, 2002). Caspases are constitutively expressed in their inactive zymogen form. Following proteolytic cleavage and activation, the caspases cleave target proteins at sites following aspartic residues (Muzio *et al.*, 1998). A representative model is the activation of the caspase cascade following Fas ligand binding to Fas, in which oligomerization of caspase-8 results in cleavage of the prodomain from its active subunit, and autoactivation occurs (Figure 1). The active domain of caspase-8 then cleaves the prodomain of the effector caspase, caspase-3. Active caspase-3 cleaves a vast number of proteins within the cell including the cell cycle regulators Cdc 27, Cyclin A, and Topoisomerase (Fischer *et al.*, 2003). In addition, caspase-3 cleaves various DNA-associated repair enzymes and cytoskeletal proteins, particularly the cytokeratin-containing intermediate filaments (McCarthy & Bennett, 2002; Fischer et al., 2003). As described later, cytokeratin intermediate filaments are a diverse family of proteins that generally exert protective effects within cells, preventing cell stress and apoptosis. Hence, their disassembly or loss renders cells vulnerable to a variety of insults and apoptotic processes. Beyond these considerations, intracellular pro-apoptotic proteins, such as Bax and p53, also increase in cells undergoing apoptosis. A variety of extracellular and intracellular signals stimulate Bax and p53 expression in granulosa cells of follicles (Tilly et al., 1995; Amsterdam et al., 1996; Kim et al., 1999; Zwain & Amato, 2001; Das et al., 2008; Salvetti et al., 2010), which result in apoptotic effects such as the release of cytochrome C from mitochondria, further activation of caspases, and ultimately fragmentation of nuclear DNA.

In a relatively recent *in vitro* study, transforming growth factor-beta1 (TGF-beta1) was identified as a pro-apoptotic signal to bovine granulosa cells (Zheng *et al.*, 2009). Essentially TGF-beta 1 prevented luteinization of the cells while maintaining an estrogenic phenotype. TGF-beta1 also induced apoptosis of the granulosa cells under control and FSH-stimulated conditions. Based upon these results, the authors suggested TGF-beta 1 influences selection of the dominant follicle during folliculogenesis in cattle by controlling the proliferation and the steroidogenic differentiation of granulosa cells. However, whether or not TGF-beta1 can be truly ascribed a pro-apoptotic role is debatable. It shares structural and functional properties with other members of the transforming growth factor-beta superfamily, many of which are essential for follicular growth and development in a variety of species (for an extensive review, see Juengel & McNatty, 2005), and thus possesses anti-apoptotic or pro-survival attributes.

Anti-apoptotic or pro-survival molecules in the context of follicular development and atresia are those that promote growth and proliferation of cells within the follicle, or counteract the actions of apoptotic molecules. Examples of extracellular factors include the gonadotropins, steroids, certain cytokines and growth factors. Intracellularly, there are a variety of molecules that directly counteract the actions of pro-apoptotic factors, while others utilize unique signaling pathways. Among the intracellular factors preventing apoptosis through these means are the regulators of cell cycle progression (e.g., cyclins and cyclin-dependent kinases); the serine/threonine protein kinase, Akt; an anti-caspase 8 molecule known as cellular FLICE inhibitory protein (cFLIP); and the apoptosis regulator protein, Bcl-2.

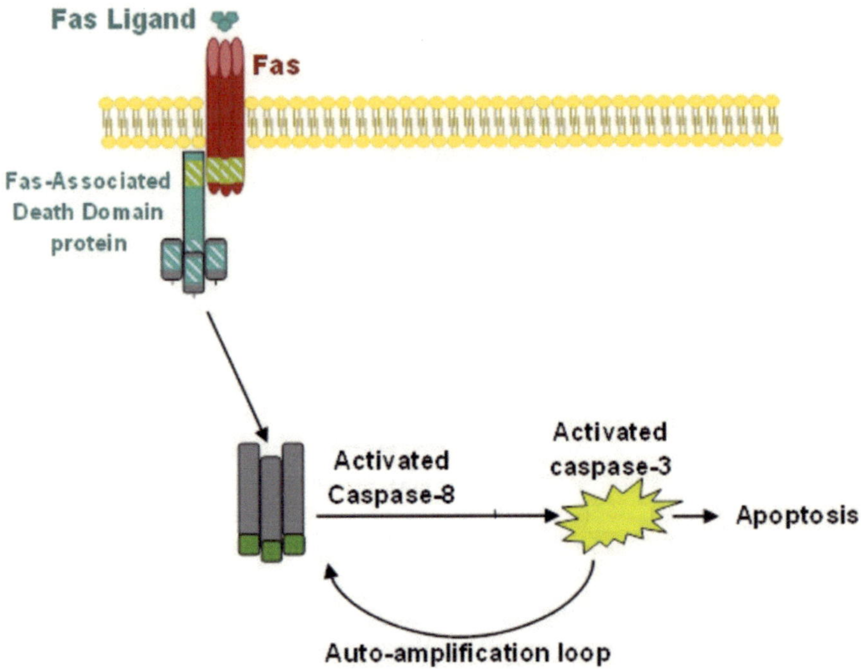

Fig. 1. Fas ligand-induced apoptosis through caspase -8 and caspase-3 activation. Fas ligand induces apoptosis by triggering aggregation and oligomerization of the Fas receptor on the cell surface. Once oligomerized, the receptor associates with an intracellular Fas-Associated Death Domain (FADD) protein. The FADD protein enzymatically cleaves the prodomain of caspase-8, triggering its activation, the activation of caspase-3, and then subsequent downstream events that result in apoptosis.

Acknowledging that growth of tertiary follicles during a follicular wave is gonadotropin-dependent, it is not surprising to learn that gonadotropins also impact apoptosis of granulosa cells during this process. In general, FSH suppresses apoptosis of granulosa cells in medium and large follices (Yang & Rajamahendran, 2000), whereas LH suppresses apoptosis of granulosa cells in large follicles only (Chun et al., 1996; Porter et al., 2001). The anti-apoptotic effects of the gonadotropins are likely attributable to their enhancement of steroidogenic enzymes and steroid synthesis within the follicle. In particular, increased estradiol synthesis is a tell-tale indication of a healthy follicle with viable granulosa cells. Quirk and coworkers (Quirk *et al.*, 2006) were among the first to determine estradiol protects bovine granulosa cells from apoptosis by increasing cyclin D2 expression and stimulating the cells to progress from the G1 to S phase of the cell cycle. As follicles progress through the pre-ovulatory stages of growth, progesterone secretion prevails over estradiol secretion as granulosa cells become luteinized, prompted by the LH surge. During this period of steroidogenic transition the responsiveness of the granulosa cells to progesterone is enhanced, triggering their withdrawal from the cell cycle (Quirk *et al.*, 2004), and anti-apoptotic effects (Quirk et al., 2004; Peluso et al., 2009). Conversely, a high ratio of androgen to estradiol within follicles is generally viewed as an indication of follicular atresia (McNatty et al., 1976; Fortune & Hansel, 1985). Although androgens (i.e., androstenedione and testosterone) are admittedly produced by theca cells as precursors for aromatization to estradiol in growing follicles; at later stages of folliculogenesis androgens have the net effects of inhibiting FSH-stimulated LH receptor expression, enhancing granulosa cell apoptosis, and promoting follicular atresia within the ovary (Kaipia & Hsueh, 1997). In summary, the actions of estradiol and progesterone within tertiary follicles may be generally viewed as anti-apoptotic and promoting follicular growth, whereas the effects of androgens are primarily pro-apoptotic, enhancing the occurence of follicular atresia.

Historically, many of the initial *in vitro* studies of granulosa cell apoptosis invariably utilized serum-containing culture medium as part of their experimental methods. In fact for some studies, serum-withdrawal during the culture period was implemented to induce the onset of apoptosis (Quirk et al., 1995; Porter et al., 2000; Quirk et al., 2000; Vickers et al., 2000). We now know that the various growth factors contained within serum, specifically insulin-like growth factor (IGF), basic fibroblast growth factor (bFGF), and epidermal growth factor (EGF), are what provide the beneficial, anti-apoptotic effects (Quirk et al., 2000; Yang & Rajamahendran, 2000; Mani et al., 2010). In contrast, other growth factors, including keratinocyte growth factor, transforming growth factor, and platelet-derived growth factor have no anti-apoptotic effects (Quirk *et al.*, 2000). Many of the beneficial growth factors likely exert their anti-apoptotic actions via enhancement of intracellular signaling pathways (e.g., Akt)(Hu et al., 2004a), regulation of anti-apoptotic genes such as Bcl-2 (Ratts et al., 1995; Tilly et al., 1995; Kugu et al., 1998; Salvetti et al., 2010), and promoting cell cycle progression (Hu et al., 2004a; Quirk et al., 2006). Another intracellular molecule known to inhibit apoptosis of granulosa cells is cellular FLICE-like inhibitory protein, or cFLIP (Matsuda-Minehata et al., 2006; Matsuda-Minehata et al., 2007; Matsuda et al., 2008). This protein is structurally homologous to pro-caspase 8, but lacks the enzymatic domain to cleave effector caspases such as caspase 3. Essentially cFLIP is a "decoy" caspase, capable of oligomerizing with other caspase 8 molecules and cytokine receptors following ligand-receptor binding, but lacking the enzymatic activity to promote downstream activation of apoptotic pathways. Among the more recent molecules recognized for their anti-apoptotic effects are the bone morphogenetic proteins, BMP-4 and BMP-7 (Kayamori *et al.*, 2009). These proteins are members of the transforming growth factor-beta superfamily and, at present, their anti-apoptotic actions within granulosa cells are attributed to an inhibition of caspase-activated DNase enzymes (Kayamori *et al.*, 2009). Thus, we are only beginning to understand the intricacies of the various growth factors and their intracellular signaling pathways as they relate to granulosa cell apoptosis, and ultimately follicular atresia. Many of these mechanisms are well-suited to hypothesis testing through molecular manipulation, for instance the use of interfering RNAs. As these molecular approaches continue to evolve, an expectation would be that considerable insight will be gained about the intracellular regulation of apoptosis within granulosa cells.

7. Influence of the cytoskeleton on granulosa cell/oocyte viability and differentiation

Beyond the above-described secreted and intracellular influences on granulosa cell and oocyte viability within follicles, there are ultrastructural or cytoskeletal influences to consider. In the last decade, for instance, a number of studies indicate the cytoskeletal elements (i.e., microtubules, microfilaments, and intermediate filaments) profoundly affect follicular growth, potentially resulting in anovulation and cystic follicles (Salvetti et al., 2004; Ortega et al., 2007; Salvetti et al., 2010). Microtubules are required for granulosa cell steroidogenesis (Chen *et al.*, 1994), but they also determine cell shape and affect cytoplasmic movement of organelles (Šutovský *et al.*, 1994). Within oocytes, microtubules promote organelle movement (e.g., mitochondria, endoplasmic reticulum, Golgi complex, cortical granules, etc.) during oocyte maturation and the segregation of chromosomes during meiotic and mitotic processes (Albertini, 1992; Ferreira et al., 2009). Hormone-induced oocyte maturation is accompanied by a surge of microtubule assembly within the cumulus cells, which constitute part of the oocyte-granulosa cell communication conduit (Allworth & Albertini, 1993). Thus it is conceivable microtubules have a similar role in regulating steroidogenesis and controlling organelle movement during granulosa/oocyte apoptosis and follicular atresia.

Microfilaments within oocytes are closely associated with the activities of microtubules, particularly the proper positioning of chromatin during meiosis (Kim *et al.*, 2000). They also help establish polarity of the oocyte, influence polar body extrusion during fertilization, and regulate cortical granule release as the block to polyspermy (Sun & Schatten, 2006). Microfilaments and other cytoskeletal components are considered essential in driving granulosa cells toward differentiation (i.e., luteinization) (Amsterdam and Rotmensch, 1987; Motta et al., 2002) or facilitating death (Amsterdam *et al.*, 1997). For instance, F-actin mediates LH-induced expansion of the cumulus cells surrounding bovine oocytes (Šutovský *et al.*, 1995), facilitating oocyte maturation and potential fertilization. Under apoptotic conditions, rearrangement of the microfilaments within granulosa cells compartmentalizes the steroidogenic machinery to the perinuclear region of the cells while directing proteolytic activities to the apoptotic bodies (Amsterdam *et al.*, 1997).

The intermediate filaments, including vimentin, the cytokeratins, and desmin, are thought to influence cell mitosis, follicular atresia, and de-differentiation of cells of the follicle (van den Hurk et al., 1995; Khan-Dawood et al., 1996; Loffler et al., 2000). These so-called "stress filaments" also participate in the maintenance of cell contact between the oocyte and cumulus cells, orchestrate distribution of organelles throughout the cytoplasm of the oocyte, and possibly control resumption of its meiotic division (Gall *et al.*, 1992), in part by influencing cumulus expansion (Šutovský *et al.*, 1995). Most recently, we have identified intermediate filaments, particularly cytokeratin 8/18 filaments, as a possible intrinsic influence of granulosa cell apoptosis during folliculogenesis (Townson et al., 2010).

The cytokeratins constitute a diverse class of intermediate filaments that derive from a family of approximately 65 homologous proteins, forming six classes of molecules (Moll *et al.*, 1982). The cytokeratins are obligate heterodimers composed of an acidic CK (Type I: numbered 9-20) paired with a basic CK (Type II: numbered 1-8). The cytokeratin 8/18 (CK8/18) filament is considered one the most abundant Type I: Type II filaments found in normal epithelia, cultured cell lines, and carcinomas. Functionally, CK8/18 filaments provide structural integrity to cells, but they also influence intracellular transport mechanisms and signaling (Singh et al., 1994; Eriksson et al., 2009). Recently, the expression of these filaments in certain types of epithelial cells has been implicated in the resistance of these cells to apoptosis (Figure 2). Mechanisms of protection include impairing cytokine receptor trafficking and cell surface expression (Gilbert et al., 2001; Marceau et al., 2001; Ku et al., 2003), and the inhibition of cytokine-induced apoptotic intracellular signals (Caulin et al., 2000; Oshima, 2002; Ku et al., 2003; Gilbert et al., 2008). These observations are consistent with earlier suggestions that intermediate filaments regulate transport processes between the cell surface and nucleus, and influence nuclear events (Li et al., 1994; Singh et al., 1994). Hence, the proposition that intermediate filaments increase cell resistance (i.e., granulosa cell, theca cell, and oocyte) to apoptosis during the process of follicular atresia is conceptually plausible. To date, however, there has been very little exploration of this possibility.

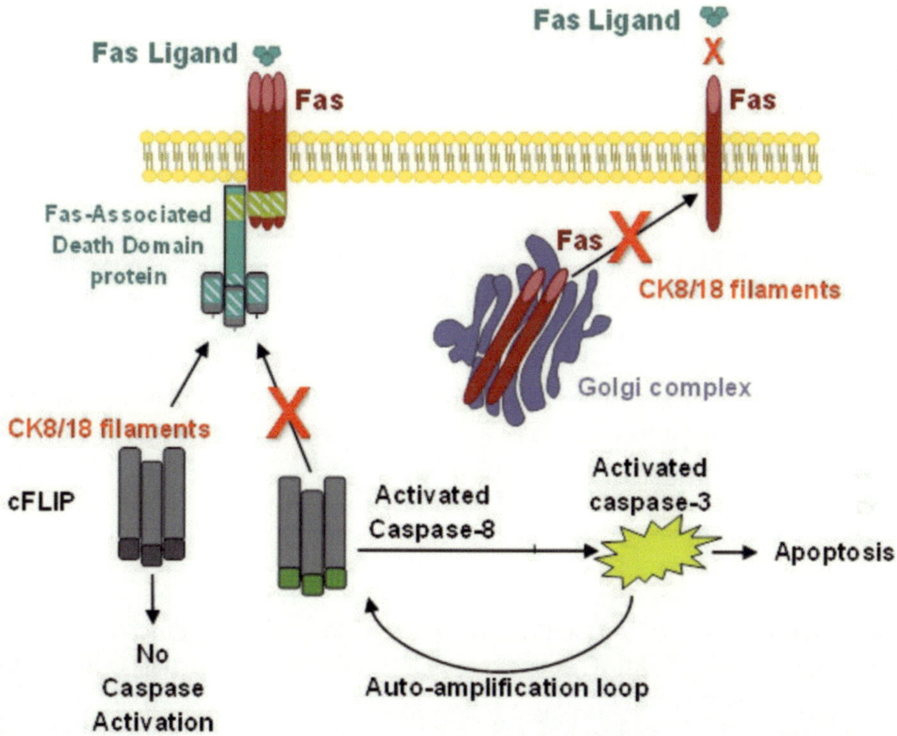

Fig. 2. Potential influences of cytokeratin 8/18 intermediate filaments on Fas ligand-induced apoptosis. Putative mechanisms by which cytokeratin 8/18 filaments prevent Fas ligand-induced apoptosis (designated by a red "X") include: 1) impeding Fas receptor trafficking from the Golgi complex to the cell surface; 2) impairing Fas receptor oligomerization and, hence, Fas ligand binding; and 3) inhibiting caspase-8 activation by enhancing the expression/binding of cellular FLICE inhibitory protein (cFLIP) with the Fas Associated Death Domain protein.

8. Role of oxidative stress during follicular atresia

Mechanistically, a balance between cell survival and apoptosis may be mediated by oxidative stress. Oxidative stress refers to a pathological state when pro-oxidants (reactive oxygen or nitrous species) are not neutralized adequately by antioxidant defenses. Cell damage may occur, including irreparable aberrations in protein, DNA, and lipid structures and functions. Reactive oxygen species (ROS) are inevitable byproducts of any cellular system in which cell division and metabolism occur. Through its developmental journey, the follicle is thus a dominant source of ROS. Several investigators have established a role for oxidative stress in cell differentiation, proliferation, and death (Ott et al., 2007; Covarrubias et al., 2008; Circu & Aw, 2010). Notably, cumulative damage from excessive ROS and oxidative stress eventually leads to cell death, hence the unsurprising relationship between oxidative stress and cell fate. But under conditions of decreased amounts of ROS, there is an early and active role of oxidative stress in evoking apoptosis; for instance, the redox status of cells (itself controlled by the thioredoxin and glutathione systems) directly modulates the initiation and execution of apoptotic pathways (Carmody & Cotter, 2001; Ueda et al., 2002; Kwon et al., 2003; Circu & Aw, 2008). Specific to follicular atresia, a few studies have postulated the involvement of pro- and anti-oxidants in influencing the fate of follicles. With the paucity of studies in any one species, below is a review of all evidence to date that investigates a potential link between oxidative stress and follicular atresia.

Past studies in systems other than the ovary have demonstrated interactions between anti-apoptotic factors (*e.g.*, Bcl-2 family members) and oxidative stress pathways (reviewed by Voehringer, 1999; Voehringer & Meyn, 2000). Bcl-2 modulates the redox status of HeLa cells (specifically the non-protein thiol, glutathione, GSH), thereby preventing any redox-dependent changes characteristic of apoptosis (Voehringer et al., 1998). Thus, Bcl-2 increases antioxidant capacity, which mitigates the oxidative stress known to provoke early stages of apoptosis. Along these same lines, Tilly and Tilly (Tilly & Tilly, 1995), using an *in vitro* follicle culture model, determined that inhibitors of ROS production and action (i.e., free radical scavengers) reduce apoptosis in rat follicles. The effects of chemical exposure (*e.g.* methoxychlor, a pesticide) on reproductive function reveal impaired follicular development, including an increase in the rate of atresia of antral follicles. Methoxychlor (MXC) reduces mRNA expression of antioxidant enzymes (SOD1, GPx, and CAT) in mouse antral follicles, and treatment with an exogenous antioxidant (N-acetyl cysteine) significantly decreases the rate of atresia induced by MXC (Gupta et al., 2006). Although the current evidence does not resolve the precise pathway(s) by which MXC induces follicle atresia, it may do so by either inducing changes in Bcl-2 followed by OS or, conversely, by leading to oxidative stress that results in Bcl-2 changes. Other chemical toxicants (cyclophosphamide and 9,10-dimethyl-1,2-benzanthracene) also induce granulosa cell apoptosis, and of relevance is the protective role of GSH in these instances (Lopez & Luderer, 2004; Tsai-Turton et al., 2007a; Tsai-Turton et al., 2007b). In ovine antral follicles, a correlation exists between an increased incidence of atresia and a decrease in GSH and the enzyme, glucose-6-phosphate dehydrogenase (G6PD), an enzyme needed for NADPH-dependent recycling of GSH (Ortega-Camarillo et al., 2009). Moreover, these changes are accompanied by an increase in protein oxidation in granulosa cells and follicular fluid (Ortega-Camarillo et al., 2009). Thus, the relative balance between oxidative stress and antioxidant capacity within the follicle has relevance to the developmental potential of follicles during folliculogenesis.

One study exploring the role of oxidative stress during follicle atresia determined that bovine follicles express increased amounts of mRNA for antioxidant enzymes only during advanced stages of atresia (Valdez et al., 2005). These findings contradict the perhaps more intuitive and widely-held perception that diminished antioxidant protection elicits apoptosis. However, an explanation for these seemingly contradictory views about antioxidants might include further consideration of the influence of follicle status (e.g., growing, dominant, subordinate), follicle size, and differing expression of each antioxidant during follicle development. For instance, in sheep, only large antral follicles (versus small) exhibit significant decreases in GSH with atresia; in contrast, another oxidative stress marker G6PD decreases with atresia in both small and large antral follicles (Ortega-Camarillo et al., 2009). In general, however, the vast majority of studies support the concept that compromised antioxidant protection is associated with the initiation and/or further progression of apoptosis.

The involvement of ROS in triggering and/or mediating follicular atresia has not been directly examined and offers fertile ground for further investigation. A recent correlative analysis failed to demonstrate a relationship between lipid peroxidation in follicular fluid and apoptosis in granulosa cells; in contrast, levels of hydrogen peroxide are increased in follicular fluid from follicles deemed non-atretic (with <10% apoptotic granulosa cells) when compared to fluid from atretic follicles (Combelles et al., 2011). At certain concentrations, ROS regulates intracellular signaling pathways, among which are the apoptotic signaling cascades. Thus, future studies focused on the involvement of ROS during follicular atresia would be informative.

The pro- and anti-oxidants described above may not represent the most upstream signals controlling follicular atresia. Rather, we suggest the aforementioned gonadotropins, steroids, cytokines and growth factors, all of which influence follicular atresia, do so via modulation of oxidative stress and, in turn, cell death pathways. Gonadotropins, for example, enhance the expression of antioxidant genes; an effect that accounts for the protective effects of gonadotropins (notably FSH) on the developing follicle. Exposure of rat ovaries to chorionic gonadotropin (with FSH and LH activity) *in vivo* increases the expression of some, but not all, antioxidants (Tilly & Tilly, 1995). The expression of glutathione S-transferase isoenzymes is increased in bovine follicles by *in vivo* exposure to gonadotropins (Rabahi et al., 1999). In the goat, granulosa cells exposed to FSH *in vitro* exhibit increased activity of catalase (Behl & Pandey, 2002). Further evidence supporting the role for gonadotropin-regulated antioxidant activity within the follicle stems from a series of rat studies. Gonadotropins enhance glutathione synthesis in the ovary (Luderer et al., 2001). FSH protects pre-ovulatory follicles from apoptosis via increases in GSH and decreases in ROS (Tsai-Turton & Luderer, 2006). Glutamate cysteine ligase (GCL), an enzyme essential for the *de novo* synthesis of GSH, is expressed only in granulosa cells of healthy follicles, and generally only following the gonadotropin surge *in vivo*, or after treatment with exogenous chorionic gonadotropin (Luderer et al., 2003; Tsai-Turton & Luderer, 2005). And lastly, stimulation of GSH synthesis and GCL expression in granulosa cells and small antral follicles are maximal following concomitant exposure to FSH and estradiol, rather than each hormone alone (Hoang et al., 2009). Overexpression of GCL in a line of human granulosa tumor cells increases GSH production and protects the cells from oxidative stress-induced cell death (Cortes-Wanstreet et al., 2009). For these reasons, we suggest gonadotropins influence granulosa cell apoptosis, and thus follicular atresia, through oxidative stress mechanisms (Figure 3).

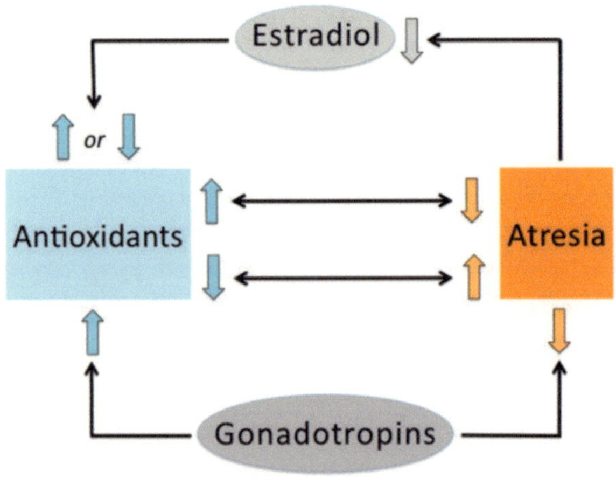

Fig. 3. Model of interactions between antioxidants, atresia, estradiol, and gonadotropins within the developing follicle. Double-headed arrows reflect correlations between antioxidants and atresia, with color-coded block arrows indicating increases or decreases in one of the parameters.

Estradiol is another hormone pertinent to the discussion of follicular atresia and oxidative stress pathways because it also influences the expression of antioxidants. In myocardiac cells, estradiol upregulates the GSH/glutaredoxin system, in turn, modulating the redox state. Consequently, the Akt/protein kinase B redox-sensitive enzyme is activated, thereby protecting cells from apoptosis (Murata et al., 2003; Urata et al., 2006). Other evidence in which estradiol favorably influences the expression of antioxidant enzymes include *in vitro* studies using cultured cells of various types (e.g., human endometrial stromal cells, vascular smooth muscle cells, mammary gland tumor cells, and ovine granulosa cells) wherein estradiol increases select antioxidant enzymes (Sugino et al., 2000; Strehlow et al., 2003; Borras et al., 2005; Basini et al., 2006). Of relevance to the ovary and follicular atresia, estradiol protects ovine and porcine granulosa cells from oxidative stress (hydrogen peroxide)-induced cell death (Lund et al., 1999; Murdoch, 1998).

As described previously, atretic follicles synthesize and contain less estradiol than their healthy counterparts. Considering the positive attributes of estradiol with respect to antioxidants and antioxidant activity, one would presume less estradiol equates with compromised antioxidant defense mechanisms of the follicle and possibly greater vulnerability to cell apoptosis and follicle atresia. However, the precise relationships between estradiol action and antioxidant activity within the follicle remain to be fully established. In bovine follicles that have established dominance, estradiol inhibits SOD activity (Valdez et al., 2005). In human follicles there is a positive correlation between estradiol concentration and total antioxidant capacity (Appasamy et al., 2008). However, estradiol is also associated with decreased, rather than increased, antioxidant expression in follicles in certain instances (Al-Gubory et al., 2008). Others have demonstrated both pro- and anti-oxidant effects (Nathan & Chaudhuri, 1998; Thibodeau et al., 2002). Collectively, these observations justify the need for further insight about the relationship between estradiol and antioxidants during the process of follicular atresia. The regulatory loops are likely complex considering antioxidants themselves may affect estrogen production within the follicle. In at least one study, SOD exposure of granulosa cells decreased aromatase activity and estradiol production despite FSH stimulation (LaPolt & Hong, 1995). Thus, a conceptual map of the specific role(s) of estradiol, pro-oxidants, and antioxidants during follicle atresia *in vivo* awaits further study (Figure 3).

Similar to the postulated actions of estradiol, growth factors upregulate the expression of antioxidants and provide protection against oxidative stress-induced cell death in chondrocytes (Jallali et al., 2007) and placental endothelial cells (Liu et al., 2010). In light of the prominent involvement of growth factors in follicular fate (section 6 above), future studies focused on the modulation of oxidative stress by growth factors, notably during follicular atresia, are needed.

In conclusion, there is growing evidence indicating involvement of oxidative stress mechanisms in follicular atresia although the precise role(s) of these mechanisms remain unclear (Figure 3). Control of follicular atresia is clearly multi-faceted and complex. Further complicating our ability to decipher the effects of oxidative stress on atresia are the dual roles of ROS. For instance, ROS may either act positively or negatively on a cellular process, including cell proliferation and death (Hernandez-Garcia et al., 2010; Poli et al., 2004). Moreover, atresia is a developmental process occurring along a temporal continuum; it is not a sudden process, and the timing of when follicles are experimentally analyzed during atresia might impact the determination of oxidative status. Such dynamic relationships are observed following ovarian exposure to MXC: increases followed by decreases in antioxidant enzyme expression occur prior to the time follicular atresia is evident (Gupta et al., 2006). In an initial attempt for protection, the follicle may first respond to an insult or its atretic fate by upregulating antioxidants. However, beyond the point of no return, an eventual decrease in antioxidants may occur allowing follicular loss to follow.

9. Involvement of immune cells and immune mediators in follicular fate

Immune cells play a key role in both innate and acquired immunity throughout the body, but they also maintain tissue homeostasis in a variety of organs, including the ovary, through cytokine secretion and remodeling capabilities. In the context of folliculogenesis, macrophages will be the primary focus of discussion here because they are arguably the most abundant type of immune cell residing within the ovary (Best et al., 1996; Takaya et al., 1997). Their proximity to healthy follicles and distribution throughout ovarian function suggests they directly impact follicular growth and atresia (Wu *et al.*, 2004). Macrophages secrete many of the aforementioned cytokines and growth factors, including TNF, bFGF, IGF, and EGF, which stimulate granulosa cell proliferation, suppress apoptosis, and promote follicular development. Moreover, in a number of rodent models, experimental induction of a paucity of ovarian macrophages has detrimental effects on follicle development and ovulation rate (Van der Hoek *et al.*, 2000), ovarian vascularization (Turner *et al.*, 2011), and fertility (Cohen *et al.*, 1997). Others have noted there are no direct interactions between macrophages and primordial follicles during the earliest phases of follicular growth, indicating early growth of follicles occurs independently of macrophage influences (Wu *et al.*, 2004). Hence, there is little debate that macrophages impact the growth and development of follicles, but lingering questions remain as to what prompts macrophage recruitment to the larger growing follicles, and the relative importance of macrophages to follicular growth in monovulatory species such as the cow and the human female.

With respect to follicular atresia, macrophages are found within the granulosa cell layer of bovine follicles only in the most advanced stages of atresia, basal atresia, in which the basal lamina has been disrupted (Irving-Rodgers *et al.*, 2001). Similar observations have been made in rodents (Petrovska *et al.*, 1996). Considering macrophages are known to eliminate dying cells and cellular debris via phagocytosis, it is thought they participate in these same activities during granulosa cell apoptosis, once follicular atresia is underway (Takaya *et al.*, 1997). Conversely, recognizing that macrophages, once activated, have a repertoire of cytokines, growth factors, and destructive metabolites at their disposal to initiate cell death, it is plausible they may play a larger role in initiating apoptosis of granulosa cells, thus provoking follicular atresia. Whether macrophages play a role as instigator, facilitator, or follower of granulosa cell apoptosis is currently unclear, but offers opportunity for future investigation in understanding their influence on follicular fate.

10. Relationship between follicular atresia and the oocyte

The follicle nurtures and supports the development of the oocyte through all stages, and it is thus pertinent to consider the potential role of the oocyte in the control of atresia as well as the effects of atresia on the oocyte. The early stages of follicular growth (primordial and primary follicles) are when oocyte loss is likely responsible for follicular loss (Markstrom et al., 2002; Depalo et al., 2003). Throughout follicular development the support from somatic cells is essential to oocyte development, but likewise, the somatic cells are dependent upon support from the oocyte. Indeed, the oocyte controls many facets of granulosa cell activities (Mermillod et al., 2008), including, ostensibly, the process of apoptosis. One hypothesis is that oocytes retaining an intrinsically compromised differentiation state may fail to support follicular development or to protect cells from apoptosis adequately. The potential role of the oocyte in modulating the selection pressure placed on the growing follicle merits experimental exploration. Whether there exists any link between granulosa cell apoptosis and oocyte quality is a fundamental question with no clear answers to date. However, current evidence supports three potential scenarios for a relationship between granulosa cell fate and oocyte quality that vary depending on the level of atresia. All three of these scenarios are biologically relevant because atresia is not a sudden, coordinated process, but rather one that proceeds progressively. Firstly, there may be no detriments of granulosa cell apoptosis on oocyte quality. This was first demonstrated in the sheep, wherein oocytes from small atretric follicles retain the ability to yield blastocysts *in vitro* (Moor & Trounson, 1977). Conversely, there are detriments to the oocyte (as manifested by degenerative changes) in late stage atretic follicles with high levels of apoptotic granulosa cells (Blondin & Sirard, 1995; de Wit et al., 2000; Feng et al., 2007; Zeuner et al., 2003). Nevertheless, follicles with a high degree of atresia, as evidenced by apoptosis of the membrane granulosa and cumulus-oocyte-complex (COC), still have the capacity to result in embryonic development (Hagemann et al., 1999). It is conceivable that the COC may be affected last by cell death in these instances (Blondin & Sirard, 1995). Thirdly, a prescribed level of atresia may impart improvements in oocyte quality, as described in the following paragraph. This is evident for oocytes originating from follicles with some degree of granulosa cell apoptosis.

It is particularly interesting that follicles in the early stages of atresia contain oocytes of superior developmental competence (i.e., the ability to support embryonic development). Blondin and Sirard (Blondin & Sirard, 1995) showed that COCs from slightly atretic follicles yielded oocytes with greater developmental competence compared to COCs from nonatretic follicles. In the case of bovine oocytes collected *in vivo* from subordinate follicles in growing, static, and regressing phases, oocytes from early atretic follicles (i.e., regressing) are of improved developmental competence compared to non-atretic follicles (i.e., growing) (Salamone et al., 1999). Furthermore, storage of bovine ovaries for 4 hours post-mortem (*versus* shorter or longer periods of time) yields oocytes with significantly greater developmental competence (Blondin et al., 1997). In this scenario, early atresia might have been induced in the follicles by storing the ovaries for 4 hours, in turn, permitting the penultimate phases of oocyte development to occur.

Pre-maturation refers to a set of cytoplasmic and molecular changes in the oocyte during the final pre-ovulatory stages of development of the dominant follicle (Dieleman et al., 2002; Sirard et al., 2006). Follicles in which some apoptosis has occurred may mimic changes that normally take place during pre-maturation, allowing the oocytes to complete their developmental program. In contrast, oocytes from non-atretic follicles may be hindered and not undergo final cytoplasmic maturation (Hendriksen et al., 2000). Several groups of investigators have documented additional evidence of a relationship between low levels of follicular atresia and increased developmental competency of the oocyte (some of which include the use of a powerful single *in vitro* production system) (Vassena et al., 2003; de Wit et al., 2000; Feng et al., 2007).

Although initially unexpected, the co-existence of an oocyte of superior quality in an early atretic environment can also be rationalized, especially in light of our current understanding of developmental competence. The acquisition of complete developmental competence occurs late during folliculogenesis, a time when apoptotic changes may have already occurred. There is evidence supporting the hypothesis that similar cellular and biochemical changes occur in the follicular microenvironment during both pre-ovulatory development and early atresia of follicles. For instance, a rapid decline in follicular estradiol, and increases in androgen, progesterone, and prostaglandin are all post-LH-surge events of pre-ovulatory follicles, which also occur in follicles undergoing follicular atresia (Kruip & Dieleman, 1982; Kruip & Dieleman, 1985; Kruip & Dieleman, 1989). Additional events common to both pre-ovulatory and early atretic follicles include the mucification of the cumulus cells (i.e., cumulus cell expansion), and structural changes in the oocyte (nuclear modifications and organelle rearrangements) (Assey et al., 1994; Blondin & Sirard, 1995). Collectively, these observations indicate there is relevance to considering the relationship between follicular atresia and oocyte quality together. Noteworthy is the difficulty of studies that aim to link atretic status of the follicle with the developmental competence of the enclosed oocyte. The atretic history of the follicle may be more appropriate to consider if some non-atretic follicles have actually encountered episodes of early atresia followed by a recovery period. In addition, there may be a threshold of follicular atresia above or below which the enclosed oocyte may be positively or negatively influenced. We acknowledge, however, that atresia is not the only factor influencing the developmental potential of oocytes. Additional considerations include the interactions between atresia and follicle size, stage of the estrous cycle, and morphological grades of the COC (Feng et al., 2007; Hagemann et al., 1999).

In conclusion, follicular atresia merits careful attention in the research arena, notably with respect to the influences it exerts on the developmental competence of oocytes. These relationships, in turn, are of biological and economical significance because they impact our understanding of fertility as it relates to livestock and human embryo production. Future research should focus on the differentiation pathways shared by granulosa cells and oocytes during atresia and development of pre-ovulatory follicles. Once identified, they may hold the key to improvements in *in vitro* maturation of oocytes, but also the procurement of *in vivo* matured oocytes of high developmental potential.

11. Relevance

Given its scope, it is likely that follicular atresia has a variety of biological roles although our full understanding of the process remains elusive (Figure 4). Ovarian follicular atresia is likened to the several instances during normal embryonic development when apoptosis possesses physiological roles, such as regulation of development of the nervous system (Martimbeau & Tilly, 1997). The massive attrition of germ cells prior to adulthood may offer the best illustration of a quality control mechanism for fertility (Krysko et al., 2008). A very large prenatal loss of germ cells coincides with entry into meiosis and primordial follicle formation; atresia could thus be a mechanism to assure the number of oocytes matches the appropriate number of follicle cells. Alternatively, apoptosis could eliminate oocytes harboring any chromosomal defects. Lastly, germ cells may be lost by self-sacrifice or an altruistic pathway by which the surviving oocytes acquire cellular elements from neighboring dying germ cells, as described during invertebrate oogenesis.

In the adult, proposed functions for follicular atresia include the selection of follicles containing oocytes of the highest developmental potential. Another interesting hypothesis relates to the large number of atretic follicles that retain steroidogenic activity, thereby perhaps imparting on follicular atresia an endocrine function within the ovary (Hsueh et al., 1994). The further pursuit of a thorough understanding of follicular atresia should provide insights into the biological significance of this remarkable process.

Clinically, there are mechanistic correlates that exist between follicular atresia and the pathological conditions leading to infertility, namely premature ovarian failure (POF) and polycystic ovary syndrome (PCOS) (Figure 4). POF is defined as the cessation of ovarian function (with elevated gonadotropins and reduced estrogens, similar to menopause) prior to the age of 40 (Conway, 2000). Its etiology is typically unknown, and the known causes of POF present a complex picture (Cordts et al., 2011). When mutated, several genes may result in POF, including the androgen receptor (AR) and forkhead box family of transcription factors (FOXO3a, FOXL2). A cessation of ovarian activity with a depleted follicle pool may stem from a reduced size of the follicle pool and/or an accelerated rate of follicular loss by atresia. The AR knockout mouse exhibits a POF phenotype together with a significant increase in follicular atresia (Hu et al., 2004b; Shiina et al., 2006; Sen & Hammes, 2010). The *Foxo3a* and *Foxl2* mutations are characterized by an accelerated rate of follicular initiation, and a follicular loss that leads to POF (Castrillon et al., 2003; Schmidt et al., 2004). Besides a spontaneous onset, POF also occurs following cancer treatment (Stroud et al., 2009), and mastering the genes that regulate apoptosis offers promise in the development of therapeutic strategies to combat POF.

Follicular atresia is also pertinent to the pathogenesis of PCOS. Many defects arise in PCOS patients, primarily chronic anovulation and hyperandrogenism (Matalliotakis et al., 2006). The primary defect is at the level of the ovary, particularly at the level of folliculogenesis,

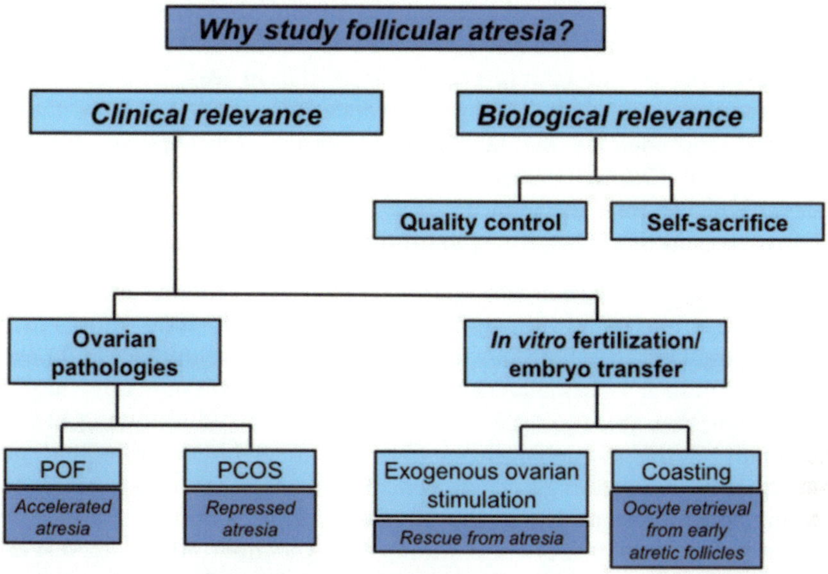

Fig. 4. The importance of studying follicular atresia.
Schematic summarizing the clinical and biological situations when follicle atresia appears involved. Further details and supporting evidence are presented in the text.

wherein the ovary contains many small antral follicles (at least more than 10 follicles between 2-8 mm in diameter). These follicles are arrested in development and do not show overt signs of atresia. The upregulation of anti-apoptotic and survival factors are hypothesized to account for the accumulation of small antral follicles (Homburg & Amsterdam, 1998); whereas the lack of developmental progression is explained by the abnormal endocrine environment in PCOS patients, notably FSH suppression (Matalliotakis et al., 2006). PCOS is thus a unique pathology deviating significantly from the normally concomitant occurrence of developmental arrest and atresia of the follicle. Indeed, PCOS is characterized by premature growth arrest without atresia. PCOS could then be considered a syndrome of repressed atresia because follicles persist despite low FSH concentrations. However, the specific aspects of apoptotic control in PCOS pathogenesis require further experimental support. Current lines of evidence support the role of a survival/apoptotic balance as one of likely multiple mechanisms explaining PCOS symptoms. Intrinsic abnormalities in folliculogenesis, notably in preantral follicles, characterize PCOS (Franks et al., 2008). A larger than typical reserve of small preantral follicles (primordial and primary) could be attributed to diminished follicle loss by atresia (Webber et al., 2003). In support of this scenario, *in vitro* cultured preantral follicles from polycystic ovaries have a decreased rate of follicle loss and an increased rate of follicle survival (Webber et al., 2007). In human granulosa cells obtained from 4-8 mm follicles, apoptotic rates are decreased (and proliferation rates increased) in granulosa cells from polycystic ovaries compared to normal ovaries. In these polycystic ovaries, the levels of apoptotic effectors and anti-apoptotic survival factors were decreased and increased, respectively (Das et al., 2008). Animal models of polycystic ovaries have facilitated our understanding of PCOS. For instance, studies of polycystic ovaries in an induced rat model show low levels of apoptosis with enhanced protection at the molecular level, explaining the persistence of the follicles (Salvetti et al., 2009). Cystic ovarian disease affects cow fertility, although it is defined in this animal as the presence of one or more follicular cyst(s), at least 20 mm in diameter and remaining for more than 10 days. Still, of relevance to human PCOS are the suppressed proliferation and apoptotic rates that appear to undermine follicle persistence in cystic cow ovaries (Salvetti et al., 2010). Further understanding of the control of apoptosis at the molecular level will facilitate the identification of any defect(s) in the apoptotic pathway during PCOS; this could then open doors to future targeted therapies.

During routine *in vitro* fertilization and embryo transfer (in humans and animals), ovarian stimulation is often employed. Ovarian stimulation protocols include stimulation with FSH, thereby reducing the FSH threshold needed for continued development and permitting the effective rescue of follicles normally destined for atresia. Consequently, more ovulatory follicles can be aspirated and multiple mature oocytes obtained following LH stimulation. Undeniably, many of the rescued follicles give rise to viable embryos and pregnancies; however, the quality of a retrieved oocyte cohort is characteristically heterogeneous. With hormonal stimulation interfering with the physiological selection pressures placed on the follicle, it is conceivable that oocytes of diminished potential are retained. Perhaps such follicles, and in turn oocytes, are compromised beyond a point of no return. Very little consideration has been given to this issue, suggesting it is a critical area for future study and improvements. A goal should be to optimize conditions for obtaining a whole cohort of superior quality embryos, which would assist in the treatment of human infertility and animal embryo production. For instance, there is a dire need to determine the effects of gonadotropin stimulation protocols on follicular atresia, particularly in the human female, with the cow serving as an extremely useful and relevant animal model.

There is little evidence to indicate that follicles are destined and irreversibly committed to atresia from the start of their developmental journey since most follicles remain capable of continued development if stimulated properly. For instance, although the dominant follicle of the first wave of the cow estrous cycle is theoretically destined for atresia, it can be rescued as long as the stimulus is provided in advance of the regression phase (Fortune et al., 1991). Atretic follicles can also be rescued by exogenous exposure to gonadotropins (Hsueh et al., 1994; Monniaux et al., 1984; Blondin et al., 1996). Currently, however, we hold little knowledge about how long the rescue period may last, or how long atretic fate can be manipulated. While diminishing the rate follicular atresia and increasing oocyte yield, superovulation procedures alone do not yield more embryos than those of non-stimulated cycles (Blondin et al., 1996). These outcomes justify the need for further refinement of gonadotropin stimulation protocols.

An ovarian stimulation protocol with particular promise in the cow involves the use of gonadotropins together with a so-called "coasting" phase. In essence, coasting protocols are aimed at collecting oocytes from follicles in stages of early atresia (Sirard et al., 1999; Blondin et al., 2002). The approach is based upon the premise that early atretic follicles contain oocytes of quality comparable to pre-ovulatory follicles as alluded to previously (see above discussion in section 10). Coasting protocols thus target oocyte collection from follicles in a plateau phase of follicular growth, during which follicular atresia may be already under way and an optimal follicular microenvironment exists. Essentially the protocols entail stimulation with FSH (in constant or decreasing dosages) followed by a period of coasting for 24-72 hours with no further gonadotropin exposure and prior to oocyte aspiration. When collected at the optimal time post-FSH withdrawal (and presumably in the throes of early atresia), the oocytes possess the highest developmental potential (Sirard et al., 1999; Blondin et al., 2002). More recently, the optimal timing for oocyte collection has been narrowed to 54 hours +/- 7 hours, post-FSH withdrawal (Bunel et al., 2011). Bovine studies thus provide promise for future efforts to manipulate the atretic status of follicles *in vivo*, coupled with obtaining oocytes of optimal developmental quality (Figure 4). These approaches stand in stark contrast to current stimulation protocols in both livestock and in women, in which oocytes are collected from follicles during the growing phase, final differentiation of the oocytes has not occurred, and oocyte developmental competence is often compromised.

12. Conclusions

In conclusion, our understanding of the cellular factors influencing the onset of follicular atresia within the ovary is only beginning to emerge. Future research focusing on the mechanisms shared by granulosa cells and oocytes that dictate cell fate (i.e., growth, differentiation, death) and, ultimately, follicular fate (i.e., growth, dominance, atresia), including the molecular, cytoskeletal, and metabolic influences, should provide considerable insight. Examples of these influences include microRNA regulation, cytokeratin filament expression, and oxidative stress control, respectively. These factors, in turn, are of biological and economic significance because they impact other aspects of fertility in both livestock and humans. Once identified, they may hold the key to therapeutic improvements in treating infertility and poor reproductive performance in animals.

13. Acknowledgement

This project was supported by National Research Initiative Competitive Grant no. 2007-35203-18074 (DHT) and Agriculture and Food Research Initiative Competitive Grant no. 2011-67016-20041 (CMHC) from the USDA National Institute of Food and Agriculture. Appreciation is expressed to Brian T. Sullivan for his contributions to Figures 1 and 2.

14. References

Adams, G.P., R.L. Matteri, J.P. Kastelic, J.C.H. Ko & O.J. Ginther (1992). Association between surges of follicle-stimulating hormone and the emergence of follicular waves in heifers. *Journal of Reproduction and Fertility*, Vol. 94, No. 1, pp. 177-188

Aerts, J.M. & P.E. Bols (2010). Ovarian follicular dynamics. A review with emphasis on the bovine species. Part II: Antral development, exogenous influence and future prospects. *Reprod Domest Anim*, Vol. 45, No. 1, pp. 180-187

Al-Gubory, K.H., P. Bolifraud & C. Garrel (2008). Regulation of key antioxidant enzymatic systems in the sheep endometrium by ovarian steroids. *Endocrinology*, Vol. 149, No. 9, pp. 4428-4434

Albertini, D.F. (1992). Cytoplasmic microtubular dynamics and chromatin organization during mammalian oogenesis and oocyte maturation. *Mutation Research/Reviews in Genetic Toxicology*, Vol. 296, No. 1-2, pp. 57-68

Allworth, A.E. & D.F. Albertini (1993). Meiotic Maturation in Cultured Bovine Oocytes Is Accompanied by Remodeling of the Cumulus Cell Cytoskeleton. *Developmental Biology*, Vol. 158, No. 1, pp. 101-112

Amsterdam, A., A. Dantes, N. Selvaraj & D. Aharoni (1997). Apoptosis in steroidogenic cells: structure-function analysis. *Steroids*, Vol. 62, No. 1, pp. 207-211

Amsterdam, A., I. Keren-Tal & D. Aharoni (1996). Cross-talk between cAMP and p53-generated signals in induction of differentiation and apoptosis in steroidogenic granulosa cells. *Steroids*, Vol. 61, No. 4, pp. 252-256

Amsterdam, A. & S. Rotmensch (1987). Structure-Function Relationships during Granulosa Cell Differentiation. *Endocrine Reviews*, Vol. 8, No. 3, pp. 309-337

Appasamy, M., E. Jauniaux, P. Serhal, A. Al-Qahtani, N.P. Groome & S. Muttukrishna (2008). Evaluation of the relationship between follicular fluid oxidative stress, ovarian hormones, and response to gonadotropin stimulation. *Fertil Steril*, Vol. 89, No. 4, pp. 912-921

Armstrong, D., C. Gutierrez, G. Baxter, A. Glazyrin, G. Mann, K. Woad, C. Hogg & R. Webb (2000). Expression of mRNA encoding IGF-I, IGF-II and type 1 IGF receptor in bovine ovarian follicles. *Journal of Endocrinology*, Vol. 165, No. 1, pp. 101-113

Armstrong, D. & R. Webb (1997). Ovarian follicular dominance: the role of intraovarian growth factors and novel proteins. *Rev Reprod*, Vol. 2, No. 3, pp. 139-146

Assey, R.J., P. Hyttel, T. Greve & B. Purwantara (1994). Oocyte morphology in dominant and subordinate follicles. *Mol Reprod Dev*, Vol. 37, No. 3, pp. 335-344

Baerwald, A.R., G.P. Adams & R.A. Pierson (2003). Characterization of Ovarian Follicular Wave Dynamics in Women. *Biology of Reproduction*, Vol. 69, No. 3, pp. 1023-1031

Baker, T.G. (1963). A Quantitative and Cytological Study of Germ Cells in Human Ovaries. *Proc R Soc Lond B Biol Sci*, Vol. 158, No. pp. 417-433

Bao, B. & H.A. Garverick (1998). Expression of steroidogenic enzyme and gonadotropin receptor genes in bovine follicles during ovarian follicular waves: a review. *Journal of Animal Science*, Vol. 76, No. 7, pp. 1903-1921

Basini, G., G.L. Mainardi, S. Bussolati & C. Tamanini (2002). Steroidogenesis, proliferation and apoptosis in bovine granulosa cells: role of tumour necrosis factor-α and its possible signalling mechanisms. *Reproduction, Fertility and Development*, Vol. 14, No. 3, pp. 141-150

Basini, G., S.E. Santini & F. Grasselli (2006). 2-Methoxyestradiol inhibits superoxide anion generation while it enhances superoxide dismutase activity in swine granulosa cells. *Ann N Y Acad Sci*, Vol. 1091, No. pp. 34-40

Beg, M.A. & O.J. Ginther (2006). Follicle selection in cattle and horses: role of intrafollicular factors. *Reproduction*, Vol. 132, No. 3, pp. 365-377

Behl, R. & R.S. Pandey (2002). FSH induced stimulation of catalase activity in goat granulosa cells in vitro. *Anim Reprod Sci*, Vol. 70, No. 3-4, pp. 215-221

Best, C.L., J. Pudney, W.R. Welch, N. Burger & J.A. Hill (1996). Localization and characterization of white blood cell populations within the human ovary throughout the menstrual cycle and menopause. *Hum Reprod*, Vol. 11, No. 4, pp. 790-797

Blondin, P., D. Bousquet, H. Twagiramungu, F. Barnes & M.A. Sirard (2002). Manipulation of follicular development to produce developmentally competent bovine oocytes. *Biol Reprod*, Vol. 66, No. 1, pp. 38-43

Blondin, P., K. Coenen, L.A. Guilbault & M.A. Sirard (1996). Superovulation can reduce the developmental competence of bovine embryos. *Theriogenology*, Vol. 46, No. 7, pp. 1191-1203

Blondin, P., K. Coenen, L.A. Guilbault & M.A. Sirard (1997). In vitro production of bovine embryos: developmental competence is acquired before maturation. *Theriogenology*, Vol. 47, No. 5, pp. 1061-1075

Blondin, P. & M.A. Sirard (1995). Oocyte and follicular morphology as determining characteristics for developmental competence in bovine oocytes. *Mol Reprod Dev*, Vol. 41, No. 1, pp. 54-62

Boone, D.L. & B.K. Tsang (1998). Caspase-3 in the rat ovary: localization and possible role in follicular atresia and luteal regression. *Biol Reprod*, Vol. 58, No. 6, pp. 1533-1539

Borras, C., J. Gambini, M.C. Gomez-Cabrera, J. Sastre, F.V. Pallardo, G.E. Mann & J. Vina (2005). 17beta-oestradiol up-regulates longevity-related, antioxidant enzyme expression via the ERK1 and ERK2[MAPK]/NFkappaB cascade. *Aging Cell*, Vol. 4, No. 3, pp. 113-118

Bunel, A., A.L. Nivet, R. Labrecque, C. Vigneault, J. Belanger, P. Blondin & M.A. Sirard (2011). Cumulus cell transcriptome regarding oocyte developmental competence acquisition under ovarian stimulation in context with FSH withdrawal and basal LH in dairy cows. 44th Annual Meeting of the Society for the Study of Reproduction. Portland, Oregon.

Carletti, M.Z., S.D. Fiedler & L.K. Christenson (2010). MicroRNA 21 Blocks Apoptosis in Mouse Periovulatory Granulosa Cells. *Biology of Reproduction*, Vol. 83, No. 2, pp. 286-295

Carmody, R.J. & T.G. Cotter (2001). Signalling apoptosis: a radical approach. *Redox Rep*, Vol. 6, No. 2, pp. 77-90

Castrillon, D.H., L. Miao, R. Kollipara, J.W. Horner & R.A. DePinho (2003). Suppression of ovarian follicle activation in mice by the transcription factor Foxo3a. *Science*, Vol. 301, No. 5630, pp. 215-218

Caulin, C., C.F. Ware, T.M. Magin & R.G. Oshima (2000). Keratin-dependent, epithelial resistance to tumor necrosis factor-induced apoptosis. *J Cell Biol*, Vol. 149, No. 1, pp. 17-22

Chen, T.T., P.J. Massey & M.R. Caudle (1994). The inhibitory action of taxol on granulosa cell steroidogenesis is reversible. *Endocrinology*, Vol. 134, No. 5, pp. 2178-2183

Chun, S.Y., K.M. Eisenhauer, S. Minami, H. Billig, E. Perlas & A.J. Hsueh (1996). Hormonal regulation of apoptosis in early antral follicles: follicle-stimulating hormone as a major survival factor. *Endocrinology*, Vol. 137, No. 4, pp. 1447-1456

Chun, S.Y. & A.J. Hsueh (1998). Paracrine mechanisms of ovarian follicle apoptosis. *J Reprod Immunol*, Vol. 39, No. 1-2, pp. 63-75

Circu, M.L. & T.Y. Aw (2008). Glutathione and apoptosis. *Free Radic Res*, Vol. 42, No. 8, pp. 689-706

Circu, M.L. & T.Y. Aw (2010). Reactive oxygen species, cellular redox systems, and apoptosis. *Free Radic Biol Med*, Vol. 48, No. 6, pp. 749-762

Cohen, P.E., L. Zhu & J.W. Pollard (1997). Absence of colony stimulating factor-1 in osteopetrotic (csfmop/csfmop) mice disrupts estrous cycles and ovulation. *Biol Reprod*, Vol. 56, No. 1, pp. 110-118

Combelles, C.M.H., M.L. Hennet & H.H. Yu (2011). Follicular fluid hydrogen peroxide and lipid hydroperoxide levels in relation to the health and dominance of bovine antral follicles. 44th Annual Meeting of the Society for the Study of Reproduction. Portland, Oregon.

Conway, G.S. (2000). Premature ovarian failure. *Br Med Bull*, Vol. 56, No. 3, pp. 643-649

Cordts, E.B., D.M. Christofolini, A.A. Dos Santos, B. Bianco & C.P. Barbosa (2011). Genetic aspects of premature ovarian failure: a literature review. *Arch Gynecol Obstet*, Vol. 283, No. 3, pp. 635-643

Cortes-Wanstreet, M.M., E. Giedzinski, C.L. Limoli & U. Luderer (2009). Overexpression of glutamate-cysteine ligase protects human COV434 granulosa tumour cells against oxidative and gamma-radiation-induced cell death. *Mutagenesis*, Vol. 24, No. 3, pp. 211-224

Covarrubias, L., D. Hernandez-Garcia, D. Schnabel, E. Salas-Vidal & S. Castro-Obregon (2008). Function of reactive oxygen species during animal development: passive or active? *Dev Biol*, Vol. 320, No. 1, pp. 1-11

D'Haeseleer, M., G. Cocquyt, S. Van Cruchten, P. Simoens & W. Van den Broeck (2006). Cell-specific localisation of apoptosis in the bovine ovary at different stages of the oestrous cycle. *Theriogenology*, Vol. 65, No. 4, pp. 757-772

Das, M., O. Djahanbakhch, B. Hacihanefioglu, E. Saridogan, M. Ikram, L. Ghali, M. Raveendran & A. Storey (2008). Granulosa Cell Survival and Proliferation Are Altered in Polycystic Ovary Syndrome. *Journal of Clinical Endocrinology & Metabolism*, Vol. 93, No. 3, pp. 881-887

de Wit, A.A., Y.A. Wurth & T.A. Kruip (2000). Effect of ovarian phase and follicle quality on morphology and developmental capacity of the bovine cumulus-oocyte complex. *J Anim Sci*, Vol. 78, No. 5, pp. 1277-1283

Depalo, R., L. Nappi, G. Loverro, S. Bettocchi, M.L. Caruso, A.M. Valentini & L. Selvaggi (2003). Evidence of apoptosis in human primordial and primary follicles. *Hum Reprod*, Vol. 18, No. 12, pp. 2678-2682

Dieleman, S.J., P.J. Hendriksen, D. Viuff, P.D. Thomsen, P. Hyttel, H.M. Knijn, C. Wrenzycki, T.A. Kruip, H. Niemann, B.M. Gadella, M.M. Bevers & P.L. Vos (2002). Effects of in vivo prematuration and in vivo final maturation on developmental capacity and quality of pre-implantation embryos. *Theriogenology*, Vol. 57, No. 1, pp. 5-20

Eriksson, J.E., T. Dechat, B. Grin, B. Helfand, M. Mendez, H.M. Pallari & R.D. Goldman (2009). Introducing intermediate filaments: from discovery to disease. *J Clin Invest*, Vol. 119, No. 7, pp. 1763-1771

Faddy, M.J., R.G. Gosden, A. Gougeon, S.J. Richardson & J.F. Nelson (1992). Accelerated disappearance of ovarian follicles in mid-life: implications for forecasting menopause. *Hum Reprod*, Vol. 7, No. 10, pp. 1342-1346

Fair, T., S.C.J. Hulshof, P. Hyttel, T. Greve & M. Boland (1997). Oocyte ultrastructure in bovine primordial to early tertiary follicles. *Anatomy and Embryology*, Vol. 195, No. 4, pp. 327-336

Feng, W.G., H.S. Sui, Z.B. Han, Z.L. Chang, P. Zhou, D.J. Liu, S. Bao & J.H. Tan (2007). Effects of follicular atresia and size on the developmental competence of bovine oocytes: a study using the well-in-drop culture system. *Theriogenology*, Vol. 67, No. 8, pp. 1339-1350

Ferreira, E.M., A.A. Vireque, P.R. Adona, F.V. Meirelles, R.A. Ferriani & P.A.A.S. Navarro (2009). Cytoplasmic maturation of bovine oocytes: Structural and biochemical modifications and acquisition of developmental competence. *Theriogenology*, Vol. 71, No. 5, pp. 836-848

Findlay, J.K. & A.E. Drummond (1999). Regulation of the FSH Receptor in the Ovary. *Trends in Endocrinology and Metabolism*, Vol. 10, No. 5, pp. 183-188

Fischer, U., R.U. Janicke & K. Schulze-Osthoff (2003). Many cuts to ruin: a comprehensive update of caspase substrates. *Cell Death Differ*, Vol. 10, No. 1, pp. 76-100

Forabosco, A., C. Sforza, A. De Pol, L. Vizzotto, L. Marzona & V.F. Ferrario (1991). Morphometric study of the human neonatal ovary. *Anat Rec*, Vol. 231, No. 2, pp. 201-208

Fortune, J.E. (2003). The early stages of follicular development: activation of primordial follicles and growth of preantral follicles. *Animal Reproduction Science*, Vol. 78, No. 3-4, pp. 135-163

Fortune, J.E. & W. Hansel (1985). Concentrations of steroids and gonadotropins in follicular fluid from normal heifers and heifers primed for superovulation. *Biol Reprod*, Vol. 32, No. 5, pp. 1069-1079

Fortune, J.E., S. Kito, S.A. Wandji & V. Srsen (1998). Activation of bovine and baboon primordial follicles in vitro. *Theriogenology*, Vol. 49, No. 2, pp. 441-449

Fortune, J.E., J. Sirois, A.M. Turzillo & M. Lavoir (1991). Follicle selection in domestic ruminants. *J Reprod Fertil Suppl*, Vol. 43, No. pp. 187-198

Fortune, J.E., M.Y. Yang & W. Muruvi (2010). The earliest stages of follicular development: follicle formation and activation. *Soc Reprod Fertil Suppl*, Vol. 67, No. pp. 203-216

Fortune, J.E., M.Y. Yang & W. Muruvi (2011). In vitro and in vivo regulation of follicular formation and activation in cattle. *Reprod Fertil Dev*, Vol. 23, No. 1, pp. 15-22

Franks, S., J. Stark & K. Hardy (2008). Follicle dynamics and anovulation in polycystic ovary syndrome. *Hum Reprod Update*, Vol. 14, No. 4, pp. 367-378

Gall, L., V. De Smedt & S. Ruffini (1992). Co-Expression of Cytokeratins and Vimentin in Sheep Cumulus-Oocyte Complexes. Alteration of Intermediate Filament Distribution by Acrylamide. *Development, Growth & Differentiation*, Vol. 34, No. 5, pp. 579-587

Gilbert, S., A. Loranger, N. Daigle & N. Marceau (2001). Simple epithelium keratins 8 and 18 provide resistance to Fas-mediated apoptosis. The protection occurs through a receptor-targeting modulation. *J Cell Biol*, Vol. 154, No. 4, pp. 763-773

Gilbert, S., A. Ruel, A. Loranger & N. Marceau (2008). Switch in Fas-activated death signaling pathway as result of keratin 8/18-intermediate filament loss. *Apoptosis*, Vol. 13, No. 12, pp. 1479-1493

Ginther, O.J., D.R. Bergfelt, L.J. Kulick & K. Kot (2000). Selection of the Dominant Follicle in Cattle: Role of Estradiol. *Biology of Reproduction*, Vol. 63, No. 2, pp. 383-389

Ginther, O.J., K. Kot, L.J. Kulick & M.C. Wiltbank (1997). Emergence and deviation of follicles during the development of follicular waves in cattle. *Theriogenology*, Vol. 48, No. 1, pp. 75-87

Gosden, R. & N. Spears (1997). Programmed cell death in the reproductive system. *Br Med Bull*, Vol. 53, No. 3, pp. 644-661

Gougeon, A. & G.B. Chainy (1987). Morphometric studies of small follicles in ovaries of women at different ages. *J Reprod Fertil*, Vol. 81, No. 2, pp. 433-442

Gupta, R.K., K.P. Miller, J.K. Babus & J.A. Flaws (2006). Methoxychlor inhibits growth and induces atresia of antral follicles through an oxidative stress pathway. *Toxicol Sci*, Vol. 93, No. 2, pp. 382-389

Hagemann, L.J., S.E. Beaumont, M. Berg, M.J. Donnison, A. Ledgard, A.J. Peterson, A. Schurmann & H.R. Tervit (1999). Development during single IVP of bovine oocytes from dissected follicles: interactive effects of estrous cycle stage, follicle size and atresia. *Mol Reprod Dev*, Vol. 53, No. 4, pp. 451-458

Hakuno, N., T. Koji, T. Yano, N. Kobayashi, O. Tsutsumi, Y. Taketani & P.K. Nakane (1996). Fas/APO-1/CD95 system as a mediator of granulosa cell apoptosis in ovarian follicle atresia. *Endocrinology*, Vol. 137, No. 5, pp. 1938-1948

Hendriksen, P.J., P.L. Vos, W.N. Steenweg, M.M. Bevers & S.J. Dieleman (2000). Bovine follicular development and its effect on the in vitro competence of oocytes. *Theriogenology*, Vol. 53, No. 1, pp. 11-20

Hennebold, J.D. (2010). Preventing Granulosa Cell Apoptosis Through the Action of a Single MicroRNA. *Biology of Reproduction*, Vol. 83, No. 2, pp. 165-167

Hernandez-Garcia, D., C.D. Wood, S. Castro-Obregon & L. Covarrubias (2010). Reactive oxygen species: A radical role in development? *Free Radic Biol Med*, Vol. 49, No. 2, pp. 130-143

Himelstein-Braw, R., A.G. Byskov, H. Peters & M. Faber (1976). Follicular atresia in the infant human ovary. *J Reprod Fertil*, Vol. 46, No. 1, pp. 55-59

Hirshfield, A.N. (1991). Theca cells may be present at the outset of follicular growth. *Biol Reprod*, Vol. 44, No. 6, pp. 1157-1162

Hoang, Y.D., B.N. Nakamura & U. Luderer (2009). Follicle-stimulating hormone and estradiol interact to stimulate glutathione synthesis in rat ovarian follicles and granulosa cells. *Biol Reprod*, Vol. 81, No. 4, pp. 636-646

Homburg, R. & A. Amsterdam (1998). Polysystic ovary syndrome--loss of the apoptotic mechanism in the ovarian follicles? *J Endocrinol Invest*, Vol. 21, No. 9, pp. 552-557

Hsueh, A.J., H. Billig & A. Tsafriri (1994). Ovarian follicle atresia: a hormonally controlled apoptotic process. *Endocr Rev*, Vol. 15, No. 6, pp. 707-724

Hu, C.L., R.G. Cowan, R.M. Harman & S.M. Quirk (2004a). Cell cycle progression and activation of Akt kinase are required for insulin-like growth factor I-mediated suppression of apoptosis in granulosa cells. *Mol Endocrinol*, Vol. 18, No. 2, pp. 326-338

Hu, Y.C., P.H. Wang, S. Yeh, R.S. Wang, C. Xie, Q. Xu, X. Zhou, H.T. Chao, M.Y. Tsai & C. Chang (2004b). Subfertility and defective folliculogenesis in female mice lacking androgen receptor. *Proc Natl Acad Sci U S A*, Vol. 101, No. 31, pp. 11209-11214

Hurst, P.R., J.M. Mora & M.A. Fenwick (2006). Caspase-3, TUNEL and ultrastructural studies of small follicles in adult human ovarian biopsies. *Human Reproduction*, Vol. 21, No. 8, pp. 1974-1980

Hussein, M.R. (2005). Apoptosis in the ovary: molecular mechanisms. *Human Reproduction Update*, Vol. 11, No. 2, pp. 162-178

Inoue, N., N. Manabe, T. Matsui, A. Maeda, S. Nakagawa, S. Wada & H. Miyamoto (2003). Roles of tumor necrosis factor-related apoptosis-inducing ligand signaling pathway in granulosa cell apoptosis during atresia in pig ovaries. *J Reprod Dev*, Vol. 49, No. 4, pp. 313-321

Inoue, N., F. Matsuda, Y. Goto & N. Manabe (2011). Role of cell-death ligand-receptor system of granulosa cells in selective follicular atresia in porcine ovary. *J Reprod Dev*, Vol. 57, No. 2, pp. 169-175

Irving-Rodgers, H., I. van Wezel, M. Mussard, J. Kinder & R. Rodgers (2001). Atresia revisited: two basic patterns of atresia of bovine antral follicles. *Reproduction*, Vol. 122, No. 5, pp. 761-775

Jaaskelainen, M., A. Kyronlahti, M. Anttonen, Y. Nishi, T. Yanase, P. Secchiero, G. Zauli, J.S. Tapanainen, M. Heikinheimo & T.E. Vaskivuo (2009). TRAIL pathway components and their putative role in granulosa cell apoptosis in the human ovary. *Differentiation*, Vol. 77, No. 4, pp. 369-376

Jallali, N., H. Ridha, C. Thrasivoulou, P. Butler & T. Cowen (2007). Modulation of intracellular reactive oxygen species level in chondrocytes by IGF-1, FGF, and TGF-beta1. *Connect Tissue Res*, Vol. 48, No. 3, pp. 149-158

Johnson, A. & J. Bridgham (2002). Caspase-mediated apoptosis in the vertebrate ovary. *Reproduction*, Vol. 124, No. 1, pp. 19-27

Johnson, A.L. (2003). Intracellular mechanisms regulating cell survival in ovarian follicles. *Animal Reproduction Science*, Vol. 78, No. 3-4, pp. 185-201

Johnson, A.L., C. Ratajczak, M.J. Haugen, H.-K. Liu & D.C. Woods (2007). Tumor necrosis factor-related apoptosis inducing ligand expression and activity in hen granulosa cells. *Reproduction*, Vol. 133, No. 3, pp. 609-616

Juengel, J.L. & K.P. McNatty (2005). The role of proteins of the transforming growth factor-β superfamily in the intraovarian regulation of follicular development. *Human Reproduction Update*, Vol. 11, No. 2, pp. 144-161

Kacinskis, M.Á., C.M. Lucci, M.C.A. Luque & S.N. Báo (2005). Morphometric and ultrastructural characterization of Bos indicus preantral follicles. *Animal Reproduction Science*, Vol. 87, No. 1-2, pp. 45-57

Kaipia, A. & A.J. Hsueh (1997). Regulation of ovarian follicle atresia. *Annu Rev Physiol*, Vol. 59, No. pp. 349-363

Kayamori, T., N. Kosaka, A. Miyamoto & T. Shimizu (2009). The differential pathways of bone morphogenetic protein (BMP)-4 and -7 in the suppression of the bovine granulosa cell apoptosis. *Mol Cell Biochem*, Vol. 323, No. 1-2, pp. 161-168

Khan-Dawood, F.S., M. Yusoff Dawood & S. Tabibzadeh (1996). Immunohistochemical analysis of the microanatomy of primate ovary. *Biology of Reproduction*, Vol. 54, No. 3, pp. 734-742

Kim, J.M., D.L. Boone, A. Auyeung & B.K. Tsang (1998). Granulosa cell apoptosis induced at the penultimate stage of follicular development is associated with increased levels of Fas and Fas ligand in the rat ovary. *Biol Reprod*, Vol. 58, No. 5, pp. 1170-1176

Kim, J.M., Y.D. Yoon & B.K. Tsang (1999). Involvement of the Fas/Fas ligand system in p53-mediated granulosa cell apoptosis during follicular development and atresia. *Endocrinology*, Vol. 140, No. 5, pp. 2307-2317

Kim, N.-H., S.K. Cho, S.H. Choi, E.Y. Kim, S.P. Park & J.H. Lim (2000). The distribution and requirements of microtubules and microfilaments in bovine oocytes during in vitro maturation. *Zygote*, Vol. 8, No. 01, pp. 25-32

Knight, P.G. & C. Glister (2006). TGF-β superfamily members and ovarian follicle development. *Reproduction*, Vol. 132, No. 2, pp. 191-206

Knopf, L., J.P. Kastelic, E. Schallenberger & O.J. Ginther (1989). Ovarian follicular dynamics in heifers: Test of two-wave hypothesis by ultrasonically monitoring individual follicles. *Domestic Animal Endocrinology*, Vol. 6, No. 2, pp. 111-119

Kondo, H., T. Maruo, X. Peng & M. Mochizuki (1996). Immunological evidence for the expression of the Fas antigen in the infant and adult human ovary during follicular regression and atresia. *J Clin Endocrinol Metab*, Vol. 81, No. 7, pp. 2702-2710

Kruip, T.A. & S.J. Dieleman (1982). Macroscopic classification of bovine follicles and its validation by micromorphological and steroid biochemical procedures. *Reprod Nutr Dev*, Vol. 22, No. 3, pp. 465-473

Kruip, T.A. & S.J. Dieleman (1985). Steroid hormone concentrations in the fluid of bovine follicles relative to size, quality and stage of the oestrus cycle. *Theriogenology*, Vol. 24, No. 4, pp. 395-408

Kruip, T.A. & S.J. Dieleman (1989). Intrinsic and extrinsic factors influencing steroid production in vitro by bovine follicles. *Theriogenology*, Vol. 31, No. 3, pp. 531-544

Krysko, D.V., A. Diez-Fraile, G. Criel, A.A. Svistunov, P. Vandenabeele & K. D'Herde (2008). Life and death of female gametes during oogenesis and folliculogenesis. *Apoptosis*, Vol. 13, No. 9, pp. 1065-1087

Ku, N.O., R.M. Soetikno & M.B. Omary (2003). Keratin mutation in transgenic mice predisposes to Fas but not TNF-induced apoptosis and massive liver injury. *Hepatology*, Vol. 37, No. 5, pp. 1006-1014

Kugu, K., V.S. Ratts, G.N. Piquette, K.I. Tilly, X.J. Tao, S. Martimbeau, G.W. Aberdeen, S. Krajewski, J.C. Reed, G.J. Pepe, E.D. Albrecht & J.L. Tilly (1998). Analysis of apoptosis and expression of bcl-2 gene family members in the human and baboon ovary. *Cell Death Differ*, Vol. 5, No. 1, pp. 67-76

Kwon, Y.W., H. Masutani, H. Nakamura, Y. Ishii & J. Yodoi (2003). Redox regulation of cell growth and cell death. *Biol Chem*, Vol. 384, No. 7, pp. 991-996

LaPolt, P.S. & L.S. Hong (1995). Inhibitory effects of superoxide dismutase and cyclic guanosine 3',5'-monophosphate on estrogen production in cultured rat granulosa cells. *Endocrinology*, Vol. 136, No. 12, pp. 5533-5539

Li, H., S.K. Choudhary, D.J. Milner, M.I. Munir, I.R. Kuisk & Y. Capetanaki (1994). Inhibition of desmin expression blocks myoblast fusion and interferes with the myogenic regulators MyoD and myogenin. *J Cell Biol*, Vol. 124, No. 5, pp. 827-841

Liu, S.H., J.P. Huang, R.K. Lee, M.C. Huang, Y.H. Wu, C.Y. Chen & C.P. Chen (2010). Paracrine factors from human placental multipotent mesenchymal stromal cells protect endothelium from oxidative injury via STAT3 and manganese superoxide dismutase activation. *Biol Reprod*, Vol. 82, No. 5, pp. 905-913

Loffler, S., L.C. Horn, W. Weber & K. Spanel-Borowski (2000). The transient disappearance of cytokeratin in human fetal and adult ovaries. *Anat Embryol (Berl)*, Vol. 201, No. 3, pp. 207-215

Lopez, S.G. & U. Luderer (2004). Effects of cyclophosphamide and buthionine sulfoximine on ovarian glutathione and apoptosis. *Free Radic Biol Med*, Vol. 36, No. 11, pp. 1366-1377

Luderer, U., D. Diaz, E.M. Faustman & T.J. Kavanagh (2003). Localization of glutamate cysteine ligase subunit mRNA within the rat ovary and relationship to follicular apoptosis. *Mol Reprod Dev*, Vol. 65, No. 3, pp. 254-261

Luderer, U., T.J. Kavanagh, C.C. White & E.M. Faustman (2001). Gonadotropin regulation of glutathione synthesis in the rat ovary. *Reprod Toxicol*, Vol. 15, No. 5, pp. 495-504

Lund, S.A., J. Murdoch, E.A. Van Kirk & W.J. Murdoch (1999). Mitogenic and antioxidant mechanisms of estradiol action in preovulatory ovine follicles: relevance to luteal function. *Biol Reprod*, Vol. 61, No. 2, pp. 388-392

Mani, A.M., M.A. Fenwick, Z. Cheng, M.K. Sharma, D. Singh & D.C. Wathes (2010). IGF1 induces up-regulation of steroidogenic and apoptotic regulatory genes via activation of phosphatidylinositol-dependent kinase/AKT in bovine granulosa cells. *Reproduction*, Vol. 139, No. 1, pp. 139-151

Marceau, N., A. Loranger, S. Gilbert, N. Daigle & S. Champetier (2001). Keratin-mediated resistance to stress and apoptosis in simple epithelial cells in relation to health and disease. *Biochem Cell Biol*, Vol. 79, No. 5, pp. 543-555

Marion, G.B., H.T. Gier & J.B. Choudary (1968). Micromorphology of the bovine ovarian follicular system. *J Anim Sci*, Vol. 27, No. 2, pp. 451-465

Markstrom, E., E. Svensson, R. Shao, B. Svanberg & H. Billig (2002). Survival factors regulating ovarian apoptosis -- dependence on follicle differentiation. *Reproduction*, Vol. 123, No. 1, pp. 23-30

Martimbeau, S. & J.L. Tilly (1997). Physiological cell death in endocrine-dependent tissues: an ovarian perspective. *Clin Endocrinol (Oxf)*, Vol. 46, No. 3, pp. 241-254

Matalliotakis, I., A. Kourtis, O. Koukoura & D. Panidis (2006). Polycystic ovary syndrome: etiology and pathogenesis. *Arch Gynecol Obstet*, Vol. 274, No. 4, pp. 187-197

Matsuda, F., N. Inoue, Y. Goto, A. Maeda, Y. Cheng, K. Sakamaki & N. Manabe (2008). cFLIP regulates death receptor-mediated apoptosis in an ovarian granulosa cell line by inhibiting procaspase-8 cleavage. *J Reprod Dev*, Vol. 54, No. 5, pp. 314-320

Matsuda-Minehata, F., Y. Goto, N. Inoue, K. Sakamaki, P.J. Chedrese & N. Manabe (2007). Anti-apoptotic activity of porcine cFLIP in ovarian granulosa cell lines. *Mol Reprod Dev*, Vol. 74, No. 9, pp. 1165-1170

Matsuda-Minehata, F., N. Inoue, Y. Goto & N. Manabe (2006). The Regulation of Ovarian Granulosa Cell Death by Pro- and Anti-apoptotic Molecules. *The Journal of Reproduction and Development*, Vol. 52, No. 6, pp. 695-705

McCarthy, N.J. & M.R. Bennett (2002). Death signaling by the CD95/TNFR family of death domain containing receptors. New York, Oxford University Press.

McNatty, K.P., D.T. Baird, A. Bolton, P. Chambers, C.S. Corker & H. McLean (1976). Concentration of oestrogens and androgens in human ovarian venous plasma and follicular fluid throughout the menstrual cycle. *J Endocrinol*, Vol. 71, No. 1, pp. 77-85

Mermillod, P., R. Dalbies-Tran, S. Uzbekova, A. Thelie, J.M. Traverso, C. Perreau, P. Papillier & P. Monget (2008). Factors affecting oocyte quality: who is driving the follicle? *Reprod Domest Anim*, Vol. 43 Suppl 2, No. pp. 393-400

Moll, R., W.W. Franke, D.L. Schiller, B. Geiger & R. Krepler (1982). The catalog of human cytokeratins: patterns of expression in normal epithelia, tumors and cultured cells. *Cell*, Vol. 31, No. 1, pp. 11-24

Monniaux, D., J.C. Mariana & W.R. Gibson (1984). Action of PMSG on follicular populations in the heifer. *J Reprod Fertil*, Vol. 70, No. 1, pp. 243-253

Moor, R.M. & A.O. Trounson (1977). Hormonal and follicular factors affecting maturation of sheep oocytes in vitro and their subsequent developmental capacity. *J Reprod Fertil*, Vol. 49, No. 1, pp. 101-109

Mossman, H.W. & K.L. Duke (1973). Comparative morphology of the mammalian ovary, The University of Wisconsin Press.

Motta, P.M., S.A. Nottola, G. Familiari, S. Makabe, T. Stallone & G. Macchiarelli (2002). Morphodynamics of the follicular-luteal complex during early ovarian development and reproductive life. International Review of Cytology. W. J. Kwang, Academic Press. Volume 223: 177-288.

Murata, H., Y. Ihara, H. Nakamura, J. Yodoi, K. Sumikawa & T. Kondo (2003). Glutaredoxin exerts an antiapoptotic effect by regulating the redox state of Akt. *J Biol Chem*, Vol. 278, No. 50, pp. 50226-50233

Murdoch, W.J. (1998). Inhibition by oestradiol of oxidative stress-induced apoptosis in pig ovarian tissues. *J Reprod Fertil*, Vol. 114, No. 1, pp. 127-130

Muzio, M., B.R. Stockwell, H.R. Stennicke, G.S. Salvesen & V.M. Dixit (1998). An induced proximity model for caspase-8 activation. *J Biol Chem*, Vol. 273, No. 5, pp. 2926-2930

Nathan, L. & G. Chaudhuri (1998). Antioxidant and prooxidant actions of estrogens: potential physiological and clinical implications. *Semin Reprod Endocrinol*, Vol. 16, No. 4, pp. 309-314

Ohno, S. & J.B. Smith (1964). Role of Fetal Follicular Cells in Meiosis of Mammalian Ooecytes. *Cytogenetics*, Vol. 13, No. pp. 324-333

Oktay, K., D. Briggs & R.G. Gosden (1997). Ontogeny of Follicle-Stimulating Hormone Receptor Gene Expression in Isolated Human Ovarian Follicles. *Journal of Clinical Endocrinology & Metabolism*, Vol. 82, No. 11, pp. 3748-3751

Oktem, O. & B. Urman (2010). Understanding follicle growth in vivo. *Hum Reprod*, Vol. 25, No. 12, pp. 2944-2954

Ortega, H.H., N.R. Salvetti, L.A. Müller, P. Amable, J.A. Lorente, C.G. Barbeito & E.J. Gimeno (2007). Characterization of Cytoskeletal Proteins in Follicular Structures of Cows with Cystic Ovarian Disease. *Journal of Comparative Pathology*, Vol. 136, No. 4, pp. 222-230

Ortega-Camarillo, C., A. Gonzalez-Gonzalez, M. Vergara-Onofre, E. Gonzalez-Padilla, A. Avalos-Rodriguez, M.E. Gutierrez-Rodriguez, L. Arriaga-Pizano, M. Cruz, L.A. Baiza-Gutman & M. Diaz-Flores (2009). Changes in the glucose-6-phosphate dehydrogenase activity in granulosa cells during follicular atresia in ewes. *Reproduction*, Vol. 137, No. 6, pp. 979-986

Oshima, R.G. (2002). Apoptosis and keratin intermediate filaments. *Cell Death Differ*, Vol. 9, No. 5, pp. 486-492

Ott, M., V. Gogvadze, S. Orrenius & B. Zhivotovsky (2007). Mitochondria, oxidative stress and cell death. *Apoptosis*, Vol. 12, No. 5, pp. 913-922

Peluffo, M.C., R.L. Stouffer & M. Tesone (2007). Activity and expression of different members of the caspase family in the rat corpus luteum during pregnancy and postpartum. *Am J Physiol Endocrinol Metab*, Vol. 293, No. 5, pp. E1215-1223

Peluso, J.J., X. Liu, A. Gawkowska & E. Johnston-MacAnanny (2009). Progesterone Activates a Progesterone Receptor Membrane Component 1-Dependent Mechanism That Promotes Human Granulosa/Luteal Cell Survival But Not Progesterone Secretion. *Journal of Clinical Endocrinology & Metabolism*, Vol. 94, No. 7, pp. 2644-2649

Peters, H., A.G. Byskov & J. Grinsted (1978). Follicular growth in fetal and prepubertal ovaries of humans and other primates. *Clin Endocrinol Metab*, Vol. 7, No. 3, pp. 469-485

Petrovska, M., D.G. Dimitrov & S.D. Michael (1996). Quantitative changes in macrophage distribution in normal mouse ovary over the course of the estrous cycle examined with an image analysis system. *Am J Reprod Immunol*, Vol. 36, No. 3, pp. 175-183

Poli, G., G. Leonarduzzi, F. Biasi & E. Chiarpotto (2004). Oxidative stress and cell signalling. *Curr Med Chem*, Vol. 11, No. 9, pp. 1163-1182

Porter, D.A., R.M. Harman, R.G. Cowan & S.M. Quirk (2001). Susceptibility of ovarian granulosa cells to apoptosis differs in cells isolated before or after the preovulatory LH surge. *Mol Cell Endocrinol*, Vol. 176, No. 1-2, pp. 13-20

Porter, D.A., S.L. Vickers, R.G. Cowan, S.C. Huber & S.M. Quirk (2000). Expression and function of Fas antigen vary in bovine granulosa and theca cells during ovarian follicular development and atresia. *Biol Reprod*, Vol. 62, No. 1, pp. 62-66

Prange-Kiel, J., C. Kreutzkamm, U. Wehrenberg & G.M. Rune (2001). Role of tumor necrosis factor in preovulatory follicles of swine. *Biol Reprod*, Vol. 65, No. 3, pp. 928-935

Quirk, S.M., R.G. Cowan & R.M. Harman (2004). Progesterone Receptor and the Cell Cycle Modulate Apoptosis in Granulosa Cells. *Endocrinology*, Vol. 145, No. 11, pp. 5033-5043

Quirk, S.M., R.G. Cowan & R.M. Harman (2006). The susceptibility of granulosa cells to apoptosis is influenced by oestradiol and the cell cycle. *Journal of Endocrinology*, Vol. 189, No. 3, pp. 441-453

Quirk, S.M., R.G. Cowan, S.G. Joshi & K.P. Henrikson (1995). Fas antigen-mediated apoptosis in human granulosa/luteal cells. *Biol Reprod*, Vol. 52, No. 2, pp. 279-287

Quirk, S.M., R.M. Harman & R.G. Cowan (2000). Regulation of Fas Antigen (Fas, CD95)-Mediated Apoptosis of Bovine Granulosa Cells by Serum and Growth Factors. *Biology of Reproduction*, Vol. 63, No. 5, pp. 1278-1284

Rabahi, F., S. Brule, J. Sirois, J.F. Beckers, D.W. Silversides & J.G. Lussier (1999). High expression of bovine alpha glutathione S-transferase (GSTA1, GSTA2) subunits is mainly associated with steroidogenically active cells and regulated by gonadotropins in bovine ovarian follicles. *Endocrinology*, Vol. 140, No. 8, pp. 3507-3517

Rajakoski, E. (1960). The ovarian follicular system in sexually mature heifers with special reference to seasonal, cyclical, end left-right variations. *Acta Endocrinol Suppl (Copenh)*, Vol. 34(Suppl 52), No. pp. 1-68

Ratts, V.S., J.A. Flaws, R. Kolp, C.M. Sorenson & J.L. Tilly (1995). Ablation of bcl-2 gene expression decreases the numbers of oocytes and primordial follicles established in the post-natal female mouse gonad. *Endocrinology*, Vol. 136, No. 8, pp. 3665-3668

Salamone, D.F., G.P. Adams & R.J. Mapletoft (1999). Changes in the cumulus-oocyte complex of subordinate follicles relative to follicular wave status in cattle. *Theriogenology*, Vol. 52, No. 4, pp. 549-561

Salvetti, N.R., E.J. Gimeno, J.A. Lorente & H.H. Ortega (2004). Expression of cytoskeletal proteins in the follicular wall of induced ovarian cysts. *Cells Tissues Organs*, Vol. 178, No. 2, pp. 117-125

Salvetti, N.R., C.G. Panzani, E.J. Gimeno, L.G. Neme, N.S. Alfaro & H.H. Ortega (2009). An imbalance between apoptosis and proliferation contributes to follicular persistence in polycystic ovaries in rats. *Reprod Biol Endocrinol*, Vol. 7, No. pp. 68

Salvetti, N.R., M.L. Stangaferro, M.M. Palomar, N.S. Alfaro, F. Rey, E.J. Gimeno & H.H. Ortega (2010). Cell proliferation and survival mechanisms underlying the abnormal persistence of follicular cysts in bovines with cystic ovarian disease induced by ACTH. *Anim Reprod Sci*, Vol. 122, No. 1-2, pp. 98-110

Sasson, R., N. Winder, S. Kees & A. Amsterdam (2002). Induction of apoptosis in granulosa cells by TNF[alpha] and its attenuation by glucocorticoids involve modulation of Bcl-2. *Biochemical and Biophysical Research Communications*, Vol. 294, No. 1, pp. 51-59

Savio, J.D., L. Keenan, M.P. Boland & J.F. Roche (1988). Pattern of growth of dominant follicles during the oestrous cycle of heifers. *Journal of Reproduction and Fertility*, Vol. 83, No. 2, pp. 663-671

Schmidt, D., C.E. Ovitt, K. Anlag, S. Fehsenfeld, L. Gredsted, A.C. Treier & M. Treier (2004). The murine winged-helix transcription factor Foxl2 is required for granulosa cell differentiation and ovary maintenance. *Development*, Vol. 131, No. 4, pp. 933-942

Sen, A. & S.R. Hammes (2010). Granulosa cell-specific androgen receptors are critical regulators of ovarian development and function. *Mol Endocrinol*, Vol. 24, No. 7, pp. 1393-1403

Shiina, H., T. Matsumoto, T. Sato, K. Igarashi, J. Miyamoto, S. Takemasa, M. Sakari, I. Takada, T. Nakamura, D. Metzger, P. Chambon, J. Kanno, H. Yoshikawa & S. Kato (2006). Premature ovarian failure in androgen receptor-deficient mice. *Proc Natl Acad Sci U S A*, Vol. 103, No. 1, pp. 224-229

Singh, S., J.R. Koke, P.D. Gupta & S.K. Malhotra (1994). Multiple roles of intermediate filaments. *Cytobios*, Vol. 77, No. 308, pp. 41-57

Sirard, M.A., L. Picard, M. Dery, K. Coenen & P. Blondin (1999). The time interval between FSH administration and ovarian aspiration influences the development of cattle oocytes. *Theriogenology*, Vol. 51, No. 4, pp. 699-708

Sirard, M.A., F. Richard, P. Blondin & C. Robert (2006). Contribution of the oocyte to embryo quality. *Theriogenology*, Vol. 65, No. 1, pp. 126-136

Sirois, J. & J.E. Fortune (1988). Ovarian follicular dynamics during the estrous cycle in heifers monitored by real-time ultrasonography. *Biology of Reproduction*, Vol. 39, No. 2, pp. 308-317

Strehlow, K., S. Rotter, S. Wassmann, O. Adam, C. Grohe, K. Laufs, M. Bohm & G. Nickenig (2003). Modulation of antioxidant enzyme expression and function by estrogen. *Circ Res*, Vol. 93, No. 2, pp. 170-177

Stroud, J.S., D. Mutch, J. Rader, M. Powell, P.H. Thaker & P.W. Grigsby (2009). Effects of cancer treatment on ovarian function. *Fertil Steril*, Vol. 92, No. 2, pp. 417-427

Sugino, N., S. Kashida, S. Takiguchi, Y. Nakamura & H. Kato (2000). Induction of superoxide dismutase by decidualization in human endometrial stromal cells. *Mol Hum Reprod*, Vol. 6, No. 2, pp. 178-184

Sun, Q.-Y. & H. Schatten (2006). Regulation of dynamic events by microfilaments during oocyte maturation and fertilization. *Reproduction*, Vol. 131, No. 2, pp. 193-205

Šutovský, P., J.E. Fléchon & A. Pavlok (1994). Microfilaments, microtubules and intermediate filaments fulfil differntial roles during gonadotropin-induced expansion of bovine cumulus oophorus. *Reprod. Nutr. Dev.*, Vol. 34, No. pp. 415-425

Šutovský, P., J.E. Fléchon & A. Pavlok (1995). F-actin is involved in control of bovine cumulus expansion. *Molecular Reproduction and Development*, Vol. 41, No. 4, pp. 521-529

Takaya, R., T. Fukaya, H. Sasano, T. Suzuki, M. Tamura & A. Yajima (1997). Macrophages in normal cycling human ovaries; immunohistochemical localization and characterization. *Hum Reprod*, Vol. 12, No. 7, pp. 1508-1512

Thibodeau, P.A., R. Kachadourian, R. Lemay, M. Bisson, B.J. Day & B. Paquette (2002). In vitro pro- and antioxidant properties of estrogens. *J Steroid Biochem Mol Biol*, Vol. 81, No. 3, pp. 227-236

Tilly, J.L. (1996). Apoptosis and ovarian function. *Rev Reprod*, Vol. 1, No. 3, pp. 162-172

Tilly, J.L., K.I. Kowalski, A.L. Johnson & A.J.W. Hsueh (1991). Involvement of apoptosis in ovarian follicular atresia and postovulatory regression. *Endocrinology*, Vol. 129, No. 5, pp. 2799-2801

Tilly, J.L. & K.I. Tilly (1995). Inhibitors of oxidative stress mimic the ability of follicle-stimulating hormone to suppress apoptosis in cultured rat ovarian follicles. *Endocrinology*, Vol. 136, No. 1, pp. 242-252

Tilly, J.L., K.I. Tilly, M.L. Kenton & A.L. Johnson (1995). Expression of members of the bcl-2 gene family in the immature rat ovary: equine chorionic gonadotropin-mediated inhibition of granulosa cell apoptosis is associated with decreased bax and constitutive bcl-2 and bcl-xlong messenger ribonucleic acid levels. *Endocrinology*, Vol. 136, No. 1, pp. 232-241

Tingen, C., A. Kim & T.K. Woodruff (2009). The primordial pool of follicles and nest breakdown in mammalian ovaries. *Mol Hum Reprod*, Vol. 15, No. 12, pp. 795-803

Tsai-Turton, M. & U. Luderer (2005). Gonadotropin regulation of glutamate cysteine ligase catalytic and modifier subunit expression in rat ovary is subunit and follicle stage specific. *Am J Physiol Endocrinol Metab*, Vol. 289, No. 3, pp. E391-402

Tsai-Turton, M. & U. Luderer (2006). Opposing effects of glutathione depletion and follicle-stimulating hormone on reactive oxygen species and apoptosis in cultured preovulatory rat follicles. *Endocrinology*, Vol. 147, No. 3, pp. 1224-1236

Tsai-Turton, M., B.T. Luong, Y. Tan & U. Luderer (2007a). Cyclophosphamide-induced apoptosis in COV434 human granulosa cells involves oxidative stress and glutathione depletion. *Toxicol Sci*, Vol. 98, No. 1, pp. 216-230

Tsai-Turton, M., B.N. Nakamura & U. Luderer (2007b). Induction of apoptosis by 9,10-dimethyl-1,2-benzanthracene in cultured preovulatory rat follicles is preceded by a rise in reactive oxygen species and is prevented by glutathione. *Biol Reprod*, Vol. 77, No. 3, pp. 442-451

Turner, E.C., J. Hughes, H. Wilson, M. Clay, K.J. Mylonas, T. Kipari, W.C. Duncan & H.M. Fraser (2011). Conditional ablation of macrophages disrupts ovarian vasculature. *Reproduction*, Vol. 141, No. 6, pp. 821-831

Ueda, S., H. Masutani, H. Nakamura, T. Tanaka, M. Ueno & J. Yodoi (2002). Redox control of cell death. *Antioxid Redox Signal*, Vol. 4, No. 3, pp. 405-414

Urata, Y., Y. Ihara, H. Murata, S. Goto, T. Koji, J. Yodoi, S. Inoue & T. Kondo (2006). 17Beta-estradiol protects against oxidative stress-induced cell death through the glutathione/glutaredoxin-dependent redox regulation of Akt in myocardiac H9c2 cells. *J Biol Chem*, Vol. 281, No. 19, pp. 13092-13102

Valdez, K.E., S.P. Cuneo & A.M. Turzillo (2005). Regulation of apoptosis in the atresia of dominant bovine follicles of the first follicular wave following ovulation. *Reproduction*, Vol. 130, No. 1, pp. 71-81

van den Hurk, R., G. Dijkstra, F.N. van Mil, S.C.J. Hulshof & T.S.G.A.M. van den Ingh (1995). Distribution of the intermediate filament proteins vimentin, keratin, and desmin in the bovine ovary. *Molecular Reproduction and Development*, Vol. 41, No. 4, pp. 459-467

Van der Hoek, K.H., S. Maddocks, C.M. Woodhouse, N. van Rooijen, S.A. Robertson & R.J. Norman (2000). Intrabursal injection of clodronate liposomes causes macrophage depletion and inhibits ovulation in the mouse ovary. *Biol Reprod*, Vol. 62, No. 4, pp. 1059-1066

Vassena, R., R.J. Mapletoft, S. Allodi, J. Singh & G.P. Adams (2003). Morphology and developmental competence of bovine oocytes relative to follicular status. *Theriogenology*, Vol. 60, No. 5, pp. 923-932

Vickers, S.L., R.G. Cowan, R.M. Harman, D.A. Porter & S.M. Quirk (2000). Expression and Activity of the Fas Antigen in Bovine Ovarian Follicle Cells. *Biology of Reproduction*, Vol. 62, No. 1, pp. 54-61

Voehringer, D.W. (1999). BCL-2 and glutathione: alterations in cellular redox state that regulate apoptosis sensitivity. *Free Radic Biol Med*, Vol. 27, No. 9-10, pp. 945-950

Voehringer, D.W., D.J. McConkey, T.J. McDonnell, S. Brisbay & R.E. Meyn (1998). Bcl-2 expression causes redistribution of glutathione to the nucleus. *Proc Natl Acad Sci U S A*, Vol. 95, No. 6, pp. 2956-2960

Voehringer, D.W. & R.E. Meyn (2000). Redox aspects of Bcl-2 function. *Antioxid Redox Signal*, Vol. 2, No. 3, pp. 537-550

Webb, R., B.K. Campbell, H.A. Garverick, J.G. Gong, C.G. Gutierrez & D.G. Armstrong (1999). Molecular mechanisms regulating follicular recruitment and selection. *J Reprod Fertil Suppl*, Vol. 54, No. pp. 33-48

Webber, L.J., S. Stubbs, J. Stark, G.H. Trew, R. Margara, K. Hardy & S. Franks (2003). Formation and early development of follicles in the polycystic ovary. *Lancet*, Vol. 362, No. 9389, pp. 1017-1021

Webber, L.J., S.A. Stubbs, J. Stark, R.A. Margara, G.H. Trew, S.A. Lavery, K. Hardy & S. Franks (2007). Prolonged survival in culture of preantral follicles from polycystic ovaries. *J Clin Endocrinol Metab*, Vol. 92, No. 5, pp. 1975-1978

Westergaard, C.G., A.G. Byskov & C.Y. Andersen (2007). Morphometric characteristics of the primordial to primary follicle transition in the human ovary in relation to age. *Hum Reprod*, Vol. 22, No. 8, pp. 2225-2231

Wu, R., K.H. Van der Hoek, N.K. Ryan, R.J. Norman & R.L. Robker (2004). Macrophage contributions to ovarian function. *Human Reproduction Update*, Vol. 10, No. 2, pp. 119-133

Xiao, C.W., E. Asselin & B.K. Tsang (2002). Nuclear factor kappaB-mediated induction of Flice-like inhibitory protein prevents tumor necrosis factor alpha-induced apoptosis in rat granulosa cells. *Biol Reprod*, Vol. 67, No. 2, pp. 436-441

Yang, M.Y. & J.E. Fortune (2008). The Capacity of Primordial Follicles in Fetal Bovine Ovaries to Initiate Growth In Vitro Develops During Mid-Gestation and Is Associated with Meiotic Arrest of Oocytes. *Biology of Reproduction*, Vol. 78, No. 6, pp. 1153-1161

Yang, M.Y. & R. Rajamahendran (2000). Morphological and Biochemical Identification of Apoptosis in Small, Medium, and Large Bovine Follicles and the Effects of Follicle-Stimulating Hormone and Insulin-Like Growth Factor-I on Spontaneous Apoptosis in Cultured Bovine Granulosa Cells. *Biology of Reproduction*, Vol. 62, No. 5, pp. 1209-1217

Zeuner, A., K. Muller, K. Reguszynski & K. Jewgenow (2003). Apoptosis within bovine follicular cells and its effect on oocyte development during in vitro maturation. *Theriogenology*, Vol. 59, No. 5-6, pp. 1421-1433

Zheng, X., D. Boerboom & P.D. Carriere (2009). Transforming growth factor-beta 1 inhibits luteinization and promotes apoptosis in bovine granulosa cells. *Reproduction*, Vol. 137, No. 6, pp. 969-977

Zwain, I.H. & P. Amato (2001). cAMP-induced apoptosis in granulosa cells is associated with up-regulation of P53 and bax and down-regulation of clusterin. *Endocr Res*, Vol. 27, No. 1-2, pp. 233-249

3

Mechanisms of Ovarian Atresia Induced by Xenobiotic Exposures

Jason W. Ross and Aileen F. Keating
Department of Animal Science, Iowa State University, USA

1. Introduction

The focus of this chapter is the mechanisms of apoptosis that occur during "normal" (physiologically-induced) or "abnormal" (chemical- or pathology-induced) attrition of ovarian oocytes. One of the primary functions of the ovary is development and maturation of oocytes, which occur within a follicular structure. During fetal development of the ovary, primordial germ cells (oogonia) are formed and become oocytes when they stop dividing, and are arrested at the diplotene stage (prophase) of the first meiotic division. At this stage the oocyte is surrounded by a single layer of flattened somatic cells (pre-granulosa cells) and a basement membrane to form primordial follicles (Hirshfield, 1991), the most immature follicular stage of development. As a result, the lifetime supply of oocytes is set at the time of birth, and is irreplaceable. Association of the granulosa cells with the oocyte is critical for maintenance of oocyte viability and follicle development (Buccione *et al.,* 1990). Development and progression of a recruited follicle also requires the appropriate expression of numerous factors, including critical members of the transforming growth factor β superfamily, such as growth differentiation factor 9 (GDF9) and bone morphogenic protein (BMP15) (Paulini and Melo 2011). Characterization of GDF9 function has a demonstrated a required role in promoting somatic cells of the follicle to undergo mitosis and initiates paracrine signaling between the oocyte and the follicular cells surrounding it (Carabatsos et al. 1998; Hreinsson et al. 2002; Nilsson and Skinner 2002). The impaired fertility in GDF9 mice appears to primarily be a result of loss of function in somatic cells since oocytes of GDF knockout mice remain capable of undergoing *in vitro* maturation and progressing to metaphase II of meiosis (Carabatsos et al. 1998).

Puberty, the time after which oocytes are ovulated from the ovary and reproduction can occur, is generally between the ages of 9 and 16 in humans. Female puberty is identified as the first menstruation (menarche), which usually occurs prior to the first ovulation. From birth and throughout the prepubertal period, waves of follicular development in the ovary occur; however, all of these pre-pubertal follicles become atretic. This is important to note, because, dysregulated primordial follicle activation into the growing pool after puberty, also results in an atretic fate for these oocytes. In humans, 1 to 2 pre-ovulatory follicles develop approximately every 28 days, whereas in rodents, 6 to 12 follicles develop every 4 to 5 days (Richards, 1980). Depletion of all functional primordial follicles from the ovary is the underlying cause of ovarian failure. The average age of "natural ovarian failure" termed menopause in the United States is 51 (Devine & Hoyer, 2005; Hoyer, 2005), however, premature ovarian failure (POF) is defined as loss of the ovarian reserve before age 40.

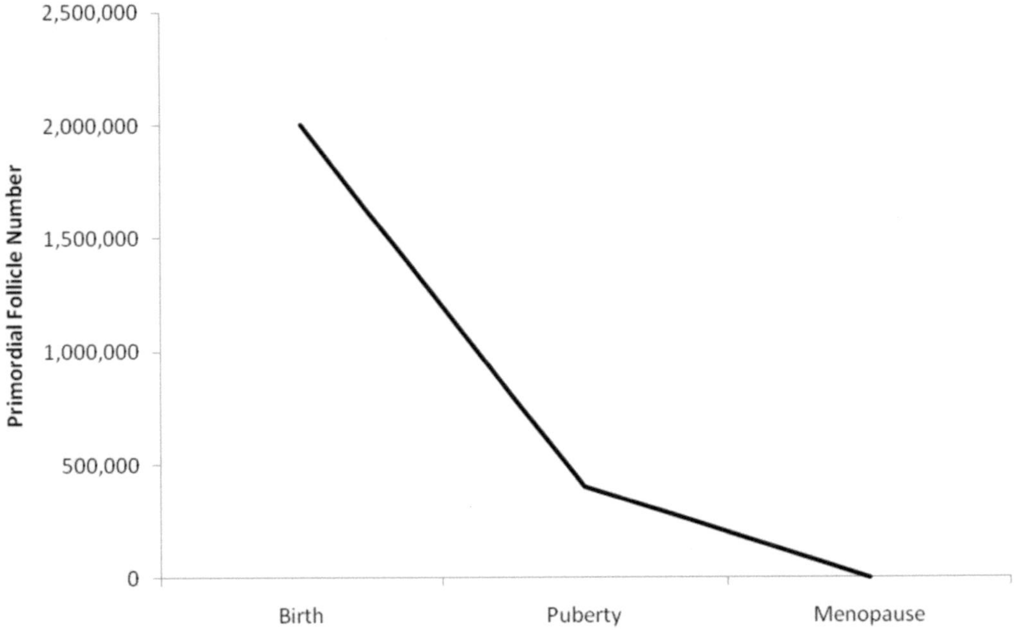

Fig. 1. Dynamics of primordial follicle atresia in humans. Primordial follicle loss at birth, puberty and menopause.

The number of oocytes present is dynamic and varies with age, with a peak in the total number of oocytes occurring during embryonic development. In humans, that number (about 7 million) occurs at five months gestation; at birth the number has dropped to 2 million; 250,000 to 400,000 at puberty; and no viable follicles remain at menopause (Hirshfield, 1991; Mattison & Schulman, 1980) (**Figure 1**). Pre-pubertal attrition of primordial follicles increases in the years leading up to puberty and the number of primordial follicles that remain at the time of first menarche define the ovarian reserve. During the lifetime of a woman, ovulation accounts for only 400 to 600 oocytes; the remainder have been lost at various stages of development by the process of atresia which occurs via programmed cell death (PCD; Tilly *et al.*, 1991). Therefore, **atresia is the natural fate of the vast majority of ovarian follicles (> 99%)** (Hirshfield, 1991).

2. Pathways involved in maintaining follicular viability

2.1 Phosphatidyinositol-3 kinase (PI3K)

The PI3K signaling pathway has recently been demonstrated to be critical for maintaining the viability of primordial follicles that comprise the ovarian reserve (Jagarlamudi *et al.*, 2009; Liu *et al.*, 2006; 2007; Rajareddy *et al.*, 2007; Reddy *et al.*, 2005; 2008; 2009; 2010). Kit Ligand (KL), a growth factor expressed in the granulosa cells of primordial follicles (Ismail *et al.*, 1996), binds to the oocyte-expressed receptor, c-KIT (Horie *et al.*, 1991; Manova *et al.*,

1990; Orr-Urtreger *et al.*, 1990). Once binding occurs, c-KIT becomes autophosphorylated, leading to activation of PI3K (Roskoski, 2005a; 2005b). PI3K are lipid kinases that phosphorylate the 3′-OH group on the inositol ring of inositol phospholipids. Activation of PI3K results in conversion of the plasma membrane lipid phosphatidylinositol-4,5-bisphosphate (PIP_2) to phosphatidylinositol-3,4,5-triphosphate (PIP_3). PIP_3 can recruit proteins containing lipid-binding domains from the cytoplasm (Pawson & Nash, 2000) such as the serine/threonine kinases 3′-phosphoinositide-dependent kinase-1 (PDK1) and AKT (Cantley, 2002) to the plasma membrane where their proximity results in their phosphorylation. Once phosphorylated, AKT can translocate to the nucleus, where it regulates a number of cellular responses such as growth, survival and cell cycle entry (Datta *et al.*, 1999). Recently, the p110 β-subunit of class IA PI3K has also been implicated to promote autophagy (Dou *et al.*, 2010) in fibroblast cells (non ovarian origin).

Mice with oocyte-specific depletion of PDK1 have accelerated oocyte loss and were depleted of oocytes 8 weeks after birth (Reddy *et al.*, 2009). Follicle destruction was determined to occur at the primordial follicle stage, indicating a role for PDK1 in primordial follicle viability (Reddy *et al.*, 2009). Downstream of PDK1, AKT has also been determined to be involved in survival of the primordial follicle stage. Mice lacking oocyte specific expression of AKT were infertile with loss of primordial follicles by postnatal day (PND) 90 (Brown *et al.*, 2010).

This pathway also plays a "gatekeeper" role in determining the entry or the primordial oocyte into the growing follicular pool (Jagarlamudi *et al.*, 2009; Liu *et al.*, 2006; 2007; Rajareddy *et al.*, 2007; Reddy *et al.*, 2005; 2008; 2009; 2010). The forkhead transcription factor family member, FOXO3, is negatively regulated by AKT. Mice lacking FOXO3 expression experienced POF due to global activation of the primordial follicle pool (John *et al.*, 2008). In contrast, when FOXO3 was over expressed in an oocyte specific manner, mice were infertile due to lack of primordial follicle activation (John *et al.*, 2008). Thus, FOXO3 has been implicated as a critical regulator of primordial follicle activation. As mentioned earlier, it is noteworthy that when primordial follicle activation is over-stimulated, that those follicles do not go onto ovulation, but are destroyed by apoptosis.

2.2 Pathways involved in follicular apoptosis and autophagy

Recently, it has been calculated that, in the pre-pubertal mouse ovary, 81 primordial follicles transition to the primary follicle stage per day, while 155 primordial follicles are lost to atresia daily (Tingen *et al.*, 2009). Thus, the majority of primordial follicles are undergoing PCD. To understand the process occurring, classic markers of apoptosis including caspase-3 and caspase-7 cleavage, PARP1 cleavage, and DNA fragmentation were investigated in mouse ovaries during the pre-pubertal transition period (PND(s) 7, 10, 13, 16, 19, 22, 26). Also, morphological examination of follicular structures was performed. These classical markers of apoptosis were detected in the secondary and antral follicles only - not in the primordial follicles. Also, no evidence of pyknosis in primordial follicles was noted. To determine if the primordial follicles were dying by apoptosis, but being cleared so quickly by phagocytic mechanisms that the investigators were missing them, ovaries were harvested every 3h across a 24h period on PND10 and stained for the presence of cleaved PARP1. Using this method, only 37 of the 155 follicles that die in a 24h period stained positive for PARP1. Another alternative theory investigated in this study was that primordial follicles are "shed" into the bursal space. No primordial follicles were found in the intrabursal space in 11 ovaries examined, thus this possible route for primordial follicle loss was discounted. These data support that primordial follicles do not die by the mechanisms associated with classical apoptosis (Tingen *et al.*, 2009).

2.2.1 B cell lymphocytic-leukaemia protooncogene (Bcl-2) signaling

Following initial recruitment of a cohort of primordial follicles, specific mechanisms are required to promote development of preantral follicles to a tertiary stage of development and then onto an ovulatory follicle. The vast majority of recruited primordial follicles undergo some form of mechanized cell death prior to achieving ovulatory status. The mechanisms of cell death can vary but are primarily accomplished through apoptosis and/or autophagy. Apoptosis (aka PCD) occurs through multiple mechanisms and can be broadly broken into caspase-dependent or caspase-independent pathways. Caspase-dependent pathways result in the activation of initiator and effector caspases that proteolytically degrade cellular components. The regulation of caspase activation is largely controlled by members of the BCL2 family, of which numerous members are expressed in the growing follicle (Yang and Rajamahendran 2002; Yoon et al. 2009), and play critical roles in cell viability and onset of apoptosis. The anti-apoptotic members include BCL2, BCL-xL, MCL-1, BCL-2A1 and BCL-w, while the anti-apoptotic members include BIM, BAD, BAX, NOXA and PUMA. The ratio of anti-apoptotic BCL-2 members to pro-apoptotic members on the mitochondrial membrane determines the atretic fate of a cell. Should they become altered in favor of the pro-apoptotic proteins, the result will be pore formation in the mitochondrial membrane, followed by leakage of cytochrome c and other pro-apoptotic proteins (Krishna *et al.*, 2011). PI3K signaling can regulate BCL-2 mediated apoptotic events. Disrupted PI3K signaling can result in release of BAD from the cytoplasmic binding protein 14-3-3 and BAD movement to the mitochondrial membrane, where it induces pore formation, resulting to the leaking of mitochondrial components, an event that leads to cell death (She *et al.*, 2005).

Characterization of Bcl-2 (anti-apoptotic) and Bax (pro-apoptotic) protein expression in bovine oocytes of variable quality revealed that while BAX expression was present in all grades of oocytes, the expression of Bcl-2 was much greater in high quality oocytes compared to fragmented and low quality oocytes (Yang and Rajamahendran 2002). This data underlines the importance of the BCL-2:BAX ratio in regulating apoptosis. To determine if BCL-2 over-expression is beneficial to oocyte growth and development, Guthrie and coworkers (Guthrie et al. 2005) created a transgenic pig that expressed Bcl-2 cDNA driven by the inhibin alpha subunit protein. Transgene expression was more prevalent in follicular cells of healthy (86%) follicles compared to follicular cells of atretic follicles (54%). Despite the positive correlation of the BCL2 transgene expression with healthy follicles, the rate of atresia or ovulation rate did not differ between transgenic and wild type pigs(Guthrie et al. 2005), suggesting Bcl2 expression alone is either not sufficient to dramatically influence caspase mediated apoptosis or that additional apoptotic pathways are contributing to cell death.

2.2.2 Mitogen Activated Protein Kinase (MAPK)

There are three major MAPK members; extracellular signal-regulated kinase (ERK), c-Jun N-terminal kinase (JNK) and p38 MAPK. The three are regulated independently, and control many processes involved in cell survival, growth, and death (Ip & Davis, 1998; Marshall,

1995; Whitmarsh & Davis, 1996). The ERK pathway is generally involved in cell growth and proliferation (Hill & Treisman, 1995), while JNK and p38 mediate the stress response and apoptosis (Johnson *et al.*, 1996; Rincon *et al.*, 1998; Xia *et al.*, 1995; Zanke *et al.*, 1996). The transcription factor complex of the AP-1 consensus site is composed of Jun, Fos and other subunits and is downstream of MAPK signaling molecules (Foletta *et al.*, 1998). As detailed in the section on 4-vinylcyclohexene, the MAPK family play important roles in ovarian follicle viability.

2.2.3 Autophagy

Autophagy is a cellular process utilizing lysosomal machinery to degrade cellular components. While not always terminal, autophagy represents another cellular mechanism of programmed cell death in addition to classical apoptotic pathways (Tsujimoto and Shimizu 2005). Screening of prepubertal rat oocytes demonstrated that while some oocytes were only positive for markers of apoptosis or autophagy, most were positive for both. Beclin I (BECNI), a Bcl-2-binding protein (Liang *et al.*, 1999), is a central protein in the autophagy-promoting complex, and has been demonstrated to be located at all stages of follicular development in the mouse, with highest expression at the primordial stage (Gawriluk *et al.*, 2011). BECN1 protein expression has been reported in the theca interna and corpus luteum in human ovaries (Gaytan *et al.*, 2008). Oocyte-specific deletion of BecnI in mice caused premature depletion of primordial germ cells and increased numbers of atretic granulosa cells. Another study found the cigarette-smoke induced follicle loss was also associated with an increase in markers of autophagy (Gannon *et al.*, 2011).

3. MicroRNA regulation of cell death

MicroRNA (miRNA) are endogenously synthesized non-coding RNAs (ncRNA) whose functional size is approximately 18-24 nucleotides long (Bartel 2004). The mature sequence confers significant biological impact on the cells in which they are synthesized and processed through perfect or imperfect pairing to the 3' untranslated region (UTR) of a target mRNA. The binding of a miRNA to its target mRNA 3'UTR generally results in posttranscriptional gene silencing (PTGS) through the action of several mechanisms, including translation inhibition, target transcript degradation and chromatin silencing via methylation (Bartel 2004; Chen and Meister 2005). miRNA are involved with numerous cell processes, including apoptosis (Carletti et al. 2010; Huang et al. 2011). Human glioblastoma cells have a 5- to 100-fold increase in miR21 and inhibition of miR21 increased apoptotic activity in these cells as measured by TUNEL staining (Chan et al. 2005). The ability of miR21 to promote cellular proliferation and inhibit cell death is a result of its interaction with several important mRNA targets such as programmed cell death 4 (PDCD4), myristoylated alanine-rich protein kinase c substrate (MARCKS) and tumor suppressor gene tropomyosin 1 (TPM1) (Asangani et al. 2008; Chen et al. 2008; Frankel et al. 2008; Zhu et al. 2007; Zhu et al. 2008). Of these three genes, all are expressed in the porcine oocyte (Whitworth et al. 2005). In mice, it has recently been demonstration that luteinizing hormone is capable of upregulating miR21 expression in granulosa cells in mice and that *in vivo* inhibition of miR21 significantly reduces ovulation rate (Carletti et al. 2010). Additionally, significant upregulation of miR21 in prepubertal pig ovaries following the development of their first cohort of antral follicles has been demonstrated along with validation of miR21 upregulation in the oocyte during *in vitro* maturation and its ability to influence PDCD4 protein expression in metaphase II arrested oocytes (Ross *et al.*, unpublished data).

4. Impact of environmental chemical exposures on follicular atresia

Exposure to environmental or occupational chemicals can disrupt female reproductive function (Mattison, 1985). A number of studies have shown that exposure to ovarian toxicants can lead to oocyte destruction (Hoyer and Sipes, 1996; Krarup *et al.*, 1967; 1969; 1970; Maronpot, 1987; Melnick *et al.*, 1990). How these effects are produced is becoming better understood and detailed for a number of chemical classes discussed herein. While outside of the scope of this chapter, it is important to note that the ovary has the capability to biotransform chemicals to more or less toxic metabolites, and these metabolism processes are highly active in ovarian tissues (Igawa *et al.*, 2009; Keating *et al.*, 2008a; 2008b; 2010; Rajapaksa *et al.*, 2007a; Rajapaksa *et al.*, 2007b) and contribute to the extent of ovotoxicity observed.

The stage of development at which the follicle is lost determines the reproductive impact. If the large or antral follicles are depleted temporary interruptions to reproductive function are observed since these follicles can be replaced by recruitment from the finite pool of primordial follicles (Hoyer & Sipes, 1996). Due to the irreplaceable nature of the ovarian reserve, chemicals that destroy oocytes contained in primordial follicles can lead to permanent infertility and POF. Also, the level and duration of exposure to an environmental toxicant can influence the reproductive impact. Chronic, low dose exposures, likely to be environmental in nature, are difficult to identify because their ovarian impact may go unrecognized for years. Ongoing selective damage of small pre-antral follicles may not initially raise concern until the onset of POF that will eventually result. Further, the age at which exposure occurs can impact the outcome. As noted earlier, pre-pubertal exposure may not cause the same extent of follicle loss as that post-pubertal, due to the higher number of follicles present during childhood. However, damage to oocytes by chemical exposures *in utero* and/or during childhood present a concern, which would not be detected until the reproductive years.

4.1 Chemotherapeutics

Concerns over side-effects of anti-neoplastic chemotherapy have increased as survival rates of cancer patients improve; currently ~ 56% overall survival rate; (Byrne, 1990). Thus, the toxic effects of chemotherapeutic drugs in women cancer survivors have become an important issue. Since the beginning of their use, the ability of these agents to produce POF has been documented. These effects have been described in patients treated with cyclophosphamide (CPA), nitrogen mustard, chlorambucil, cisplatin or vinblastine (Chapman *et al.*, 1983; Damewood and Groschow, 1986; Dnistrian *et al.*, 1983; Koyama *et al.*, 1977; Miller & Cole, 1970; Miller *et al*, 1971; Sobrinho *et al.*, 1971; Warne *et al.*, 1973). Effects of chemotherapeutic exposures on reproductive function are primarily a concern for those under the age of 40 who may wish to have children. Children exposed to chemotherapy prior to puberty are less likely to become permanently infertile than adults (Blumenfeld, 2002), however, the Childhood Cancer Survivor Study reported that 6.3% of girls will undergo acute ovarian failure, and 8% will experience pre-mature menopause (Garcia, 2007).

A time- and dose-dependent relationship between CPA exposure and ovarian toxicity in mice has been confirmed (Plowchalk and Mattison, 1992). Additionally, growing follicles have been reported to be depleted by CPA in rhesus monkeys (Ataya et al., 1989). In rats, CPA destroyed antral follicles at doses that did not affect primordial follicles (Jarrell et al., 1987). In contrast, in mice under conditions that completely destroyed primordial follicles, only partial destruction of antral follicles was observed (Plowchalk and Mattison, 1992).

Phosphoramide mustard (PM) has been determined to be the anti-neoplastic and ovotoxic form of this chemical (Plowchalk and Mattison, 1992; Desmeules and Devine, 2006). Increased TUNEL staining was observed in cultured mouse ovaries following 24 hours of *in vitro* incubation with PM (Desmeules and Devine, 2006). There was no increased staining, however, for cleaved caspase-3 in response to PM exposure, and caspase inhibition had no effect on PM-induced ovotoxicity (Desmeules and Devine, 2006). Additionally, PM induces DNA damage in ovaries of mice and rats, as detected by the appearance of the DNA repair protein, γH2AX, in the oocyte of primordial follicles, even at concentrations at which follicle loss is not observed (Petrillo *et al.*, 2011).

Exposure of PND5 mouse ovaries to cisplatin increased oocyte p63, c-ABL protein expression and TUNEL staining, all of which preceded oocyte death (Gonfloni *et al.*, 2009). p63 is a homolog of p53 that is expressed in mouse oocytes around the time of birth and has been proposed as a "germline guardian" (Suh *et al.*, 2006; Livera *et al.*, 2008). c-Abl, a tyrosine kinase receptor regulates cell proliferation, cytoskeletal rearrangement, survival and stress responses (Pendergast, 2002). Co-treatment with the c-Abl inhibitor, imatinib, prevented *c-Abl* and *p63* oocyte mRNA accumulation and further prevented follicle destruction both *in vitro* and *in vivo*, supporting a role for altered *p63* and *c-Abl* during cisplatin-induced oocyte death. Further, cisplatin increased mRNA levels of pro-apoptotic *p38 Mapk*, along with the BCL-2 pathway members, *Noxa* and *Puma* (Gonfloni *et al.*, 2009).

4.2 Polycyclic aromatic hydrocarbon

Polycyclic aromatic hydrocarbons (PAH's) are widespread in the environment from various combustion processes, including automobile exhaust and cigarette smoke. A positive connection between smoking and POF has been established (Jick and Porter, 1977). Three PAH's have been shown to be ovotoxic; benzo(a)pyrene (BaP), 3-methylcholanthrene (3-MC) and 7,12-dimethylbenz(a)anthracene (DMBA; Mattison and Thorgeirsson, 1979; Vahakangas *et al.*, 1985). These three compounds destroy oocytes in small follicles in rats and mice within 14 days following a single dose (Mattison and Thorgeirsson, 1979). A direct relationship between the dose of PAH's and destruction of primordial follicles has been shown in the mouse ovary (Mattison and Thorgeirsson, 1979).

The involvement of GSH and generation of reactive oxygen species (ROS) during DMBA-induced preovulatory follicle destruction has been evaluated. DMBA exposure increased ROS generation but did not alter concentrations of total GSH. However, GSH depletion prior to DMBA exposure resulted in increased apoptosis and cleaved caspase-3 positive follicles (Tsai-Turton *et al.*, 2006). Additionally, DMBA increases mRNA and protein expression of GST isoform pi in cultured rat ovaries (Bhattacharya and Keating, 2011), potentially as a protective measure to counteract ROS generation by DMBA.

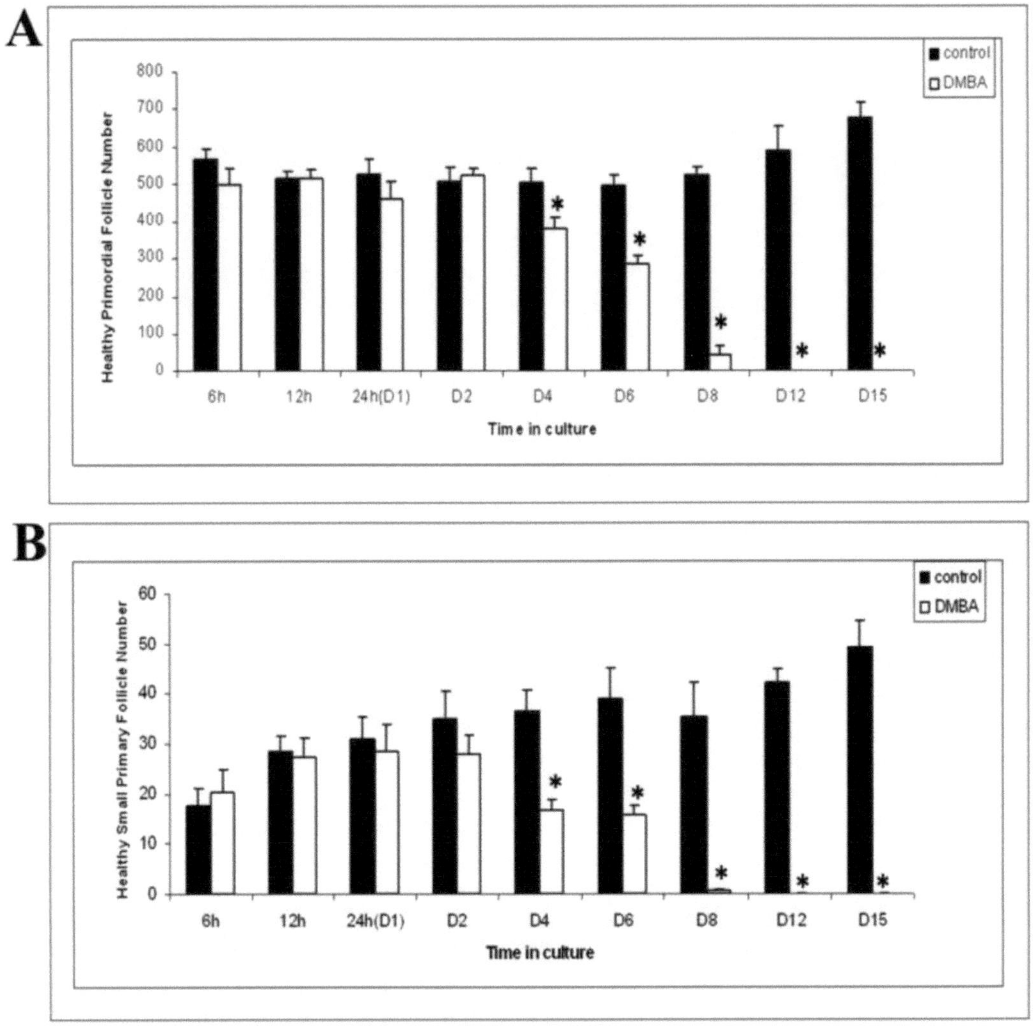

Fig. 2. Temporal pattern of DMBA-induced primordial and small primary follicles loss. Postnatal day 4 Fisher 344 rat ovaries were cultured in media containing vehicle control or DMBA (1 μM) for 2-15 days. Following culture, ovaries were histologically evaluated and follicles classified and counted. Data represent mean healthy follicle number ± SE; n = 5 ovaries per treatment; * Different from control, $P < 0.05$. Adapted from Igawa *et al.*, 2009 with journal permission.

Follicle destruction by DMBA is driven by oocyte apoptosis, followed by death of the somatic cells (Morita and Tilly, 1999). DMBA depletes primordial and small primary follicles in a dose- and time-dependent manner in cultured postnatal day 4 (PND4) rat ovaries (**Figure 2**). Up-regulation of the pro-apoptotic protein, BAX, in primordial follicle oocytes from cultured PND4 mouse ovaries is induced by DMBA exposure (Matikainen *et al.*, 2001). DMBA exposed isolated follicles were shown by immunocytochemistry to have increased staining for BAX after 24 hours, followed by increased TUNEL and cleaved caspase 3 staining after 48 hours of exposure (Tsai-Turton *et al.*, 2006). Also, ovaries from Bax-deficient mice are resistant to DMBA-induced primordial follicle destruction (Tsai-Turton *et al.*, 2006). Thus, the effects of DMBA are mediated (at least partially) by the pro-apoptotic branch of the BCL-2 family of proto-oncogenes.

Use of an apoptotic gene array coupled with Northern blot analysis identified 16 genes that were increased in mouse ovaries 12 hours after DMBA exposure (50 mg/Kg), including *p53*, receptors *Tnfrsf10B*, *11A*, *12* and *21* and pro-apoptotic *Bax* (Pru *et al.*, 2009). Immunohistochemical staining demonstrated that TNFRSF12 protein was upregulated in oocytes of follicles at all stages in response to DMBA. Some of the genes that were identified as responsive to DMBA exposure are targets of p53 transcription factor signaling. In addition, p53-deficient mice are resistant to the ovotoxic effects of DMBA (Pru *et al.*, 2009).

DMBA-induced follicle destruction is accelerated when PI3K signaling is inhibited (Keating et al., 2009). Recently, it has been determined that DMBA-induced apoptosis is mediated through down regulation of the PI3K signaling pathway (Sobinoff et al., 2011). DMBA caused a decrease in the downstream members of PI3K, Foxo3a and phosphorylated mTOR (Sobrinoff et al., 2011). Thus, DMBA induced ovotoxicity is a consequence of a number of pathways working together.

4.3 4-vinylcyclohexene

The dimerization of Butadiene forms 4-vinylcyclohexene (VCH), released at low concentrations during the manufacture of rubber tires, plasticizers and pesticides (IARC, 1994). The diepoxide metabolite of VCH, VCD, is the ovotoxic form and selectively destroys primordial and primary follicles, thus, damage caused by VCD would go unnoticed in exposed individuals. Mechanistic studies in rats have determined that VCD accelerates the natural process of atresia (apoptosis; Springer *et al.*, 1996; Borman *et al.*, 1999).

Pro-apoptotic signaling events in the BCL-2 and MAPK families have been shown to be selectively activated in fractions of small pre-antral follicles (targets for VCD; Hu *et al.*, 2001a; 2001b). Expression of pro-apoptotic *bax* mRNA along with total and phosphorylated BAD protein were increased in isolated small pre-antral follicles following *in vivo* dosing of rats with VCD (Hu *et al.*, 2001a). VCD also caused a translocation of BCL-$_{XL}$ from the mitochondria to the cytoplasm resulting in an increased mitochondrial ratio of BAX/BCL-$_{XL}$ in the target follicle population (pro-apoptotic event; Hu *et al.*, 2001a). In addition, VCD increased cytochrome c leakage from the mitochondria and activation of caspase 3 in targeted follicles (Hu *et al.*, 2001b). Collectively, these findings demonstrated a molecular mechanism by which VCD causes follicular atresia via the pro-apoptotic branch of the BCL-2 proto-oncogene family.

Activation of the pro-apoptotic branch of the MAPK family by VCD has also been demonstrated. VCD induced both JNK and p38 MAPK protein in small pre-antral follicles isolated from rats following *in vivo* dosing (Hu *et al.*, 2001b). In addition, VCD also caused an increase in phosphorylated c-JUN (p-c-JUN) protein and a decrease in nuclear protein binding to the AP-1 consensus site in the target follicle population (Hu *et al.*, 2002). Furthermore, a role for the Glutathione S-transferase isoform pi in inhibition of JNK action has been demonstrated in ovaries from PND4 rats treated with VCD. In the presence of VCD, there was an increase in the amount of JNK that was bound to GSTpi, with a corresponding decrease in the level of the JNK target, p-c-JUN (Keating *et al.*, 2010).

VCD at a concentration of 30 μM induces significant loss of primordial and small primary follicles following 6 days of exposure in cultured PND 4 rat ovaries (**Figure 3**; Devine *et al.*, 2002; Keating *et al.*, 2009). A key gene identified to be altered by VCD in a microarray study was the PI3K pathway member, *c-Kit*. When PI3K was inhibited in PND4 ovaries exposed to VCD, primordial follicles were protected from VCD-induced ovotoxicity (Keating *et al.*, 2009). It was subsequently demonstrated that VCD induces a decrease in c-KIT autophosphorylation (Mark-Kappeler *et al.*, 2011) and AKT phosphorylation (Keating *et al.*, 2011) after two days followed by a decrease in *c-Kit* mRNA expression on day 4, prior to an increase in *KL* mRNA and follicle loss on day 6 of exposure (Fernandez *et al.*, 2008). Further, exogenous KL in culture partially attenuated VCD-induced follicle loss, while there was no effect of exogeneous BMP15 or GDF9 (Fernandez *et al.*, 2008). Thus, the initial ovarian target of VCD is the oocyte, and VCD-induced inhibition of the PI3K pathway is thought to be an early initiating ovotoxic event, which precedes the activation of the classical apoptotic pathways. Additionally, it is hypothesized the VCD accelerates the entry of primordial follicles into the growing follicular pool, at which point they undergo apoptosis (Keating et al., 2009).

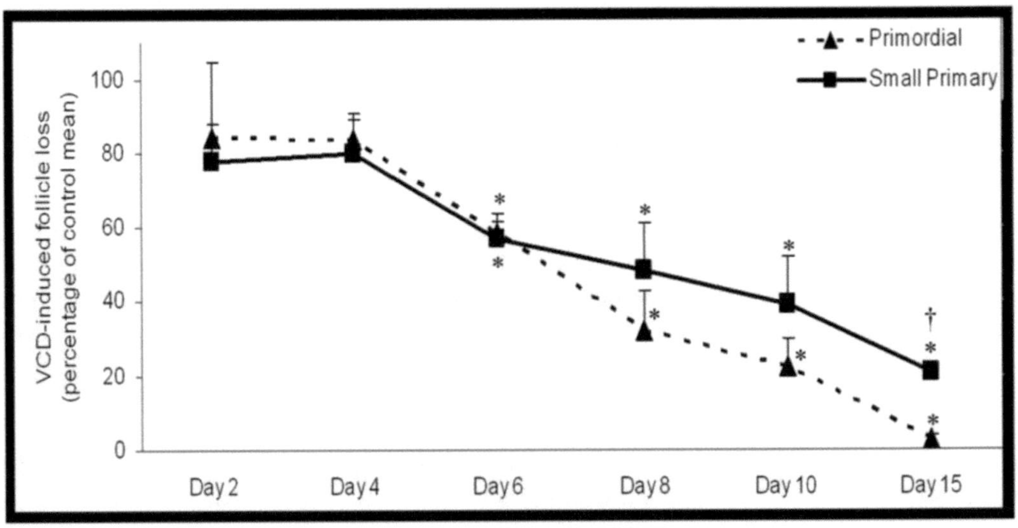

Fig. 3. Temporal pattern of VCD-induced primordial and small primary follicles loss. Postnatal day 4 Fisher 344 rat ovaries were cultured in media containing vehicle control or VCD (30 μM) for 2-15 days. Following culture, ovaries were histologically evaluated and follicles classified and counted. Data represent mean healthy follicle number ± SE; n = 5 ovaries per treatment; * Different from control, $P < 0.05$. Adapted from Keating *et al.*, 2009 with journal permission.

4.4 Methoxychlor

The organochlorine pesticide Methoxychlor (MXC) is used on agricultural crops as a replacement for DDT (Murono and Derk, 2005). Early studies reported that MXC induces ovarian atrophy in mice (Eroschenko *et al.*, 1995) and decreases steroidogenesis in rat ovarian cells (Bal *et al.*, 1984). Following MXC exposure in mice, the oocyte in the antral follicles becomes separated from the cumulus granulosa cell layer, which becomes disorganized followed by the appearance of pyknotic bodies (Borgeest *et al.*, 2002). Mechanistic investigations have indicated that MXC accelerates atresia via increased apoptosis involving the BCL-2 proto-oncogene family (**Figure 4**) (Borgeest *et al.*, 2002, Miller *et al.*, 2005) in isolated mouse antral follicles. Immunohistochemical analysis demonstrated increased pro-apoptotic BAX protein staining in MXC-treated antral follicles (Borgeest *et al.*, 2004). MXC increased *Bax* mRNA expression in cultured mouse antral follicles *in vitro* after 48, 72 and 96 hours, but decreased mRNA expression of *Bcl-2* only after 96 hours (Miller *et al.*, 2005). MXC took a longer time to inhibit growth of antral follicles from both Bax deficient and Bcl-2 over expressing mice (96 hours) when compared to the wild type controls (72 hours; Miller *et al.*, 2005). Interestingly, anti-apoptotic Bcl-2 over-expressing mice were shown to have more healthy antral follicles following MXC treatment when compared to MXC-treated wild type controls following 20 days (Borgeest *et al.*, 2004).

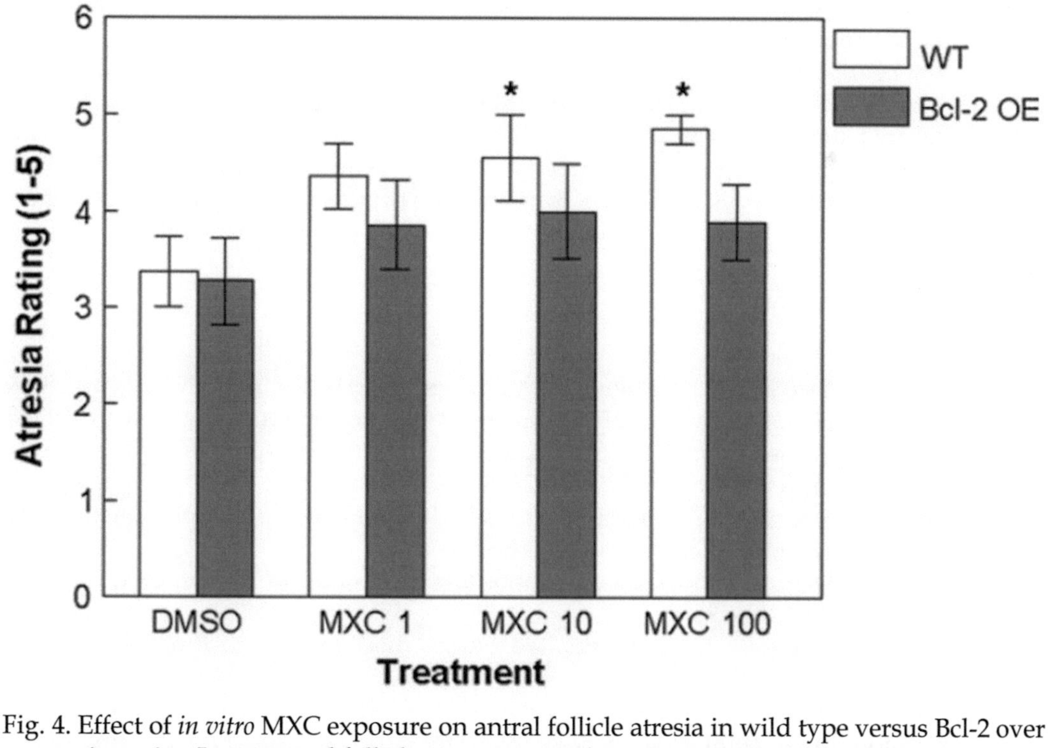

Fig. 4. Effect of *in vitro* MXC exposure on antral follicle atresia in wild type versus Bcl-2 over expressing mice. Large antral follicles were exposed in vitro to 1-100 µg/ml MXC for 96h (n = 5-11 follicles per treatment). DMSO = dimethylsulfoxide vehicle control. Graph represent means ± SE from three separate experiments; * $P < 0.05$; Adapted from Miller *et al.*, 2005 with journal permission.

Incubation of antral follicles with 17β-estradiol protected against atresia induced by MXC or the MXC metabolite, HPTE (Miller *et al.*, 2006). Furthermore, atresia was enhanced in antral follicles from MXC-exposed ERβ-overexpressing mice compared with their wild type counterparts (Tomic *et al.*, 2006). Thus, it appears that ER-mediated pathways may mediate the ovarian toxicity of MXC.

MXC has been shown to increase oxidative stress-induced mitochondrial damage (Gupta *et al.*, 2006a; 2006b). MXC-treated mouse ovaries had decreased *Sod1* mRNA and increased *Gpx* and *Cat* mRNA expression after 48 hours of MXC treatment, however, at the time of MXC-induced antral follicle atresia (96 hours), there was a decrease in SOD1, GPA and CAT (Gupta *et al.*, 2006b). At that time, MXC treatment also increased H_2O_2 levels. N-acetyl cysteine (NAC), an antioxidant, prevented the detrimental effects of MXC on antral follicle growth and atresia and the MXC-induced changes in SOD1, GPX and CAT (Gupta *et al.*, 2006b). Further, treatment with Vitamin E prevented MXC-induced OSE damage (Symonds *et al.*, 2008). Thus, the mechanism(s) by which MXC is ovotoxic appears to include an increase in production of reactive oxygen species as well as reduced capacity for antral follicles to sustain a response to oxidative stress.

5. Summary

A number of key pathways are altered during chemical-induced ovarian follicle loss as detailed in this chapter. To date, primordial follicle loss remains ill-understood however advances are being made in increasing our knowledge of how follicle atresia occurs, and the regulatory molecules involved. The delicate balance between maintaining the primordial follicle pool in a dormant state, along with controlling apoptosis and activation into the growing pool is beginning to become better appreciated. There remains, however, a dearth of information regarding which follicular/ovarian compartment that apoptotic processes are initiated within, and whether these locations change as a response to different follicle depleting stimuli.

6. References

Asangani, I.A., Rasheed, S.A., Nikolova, D.A., Leupold, J.H., Colburn, N.H., Post, S. & Allgayer, H. (2008). MicroRNA-21 (miR-21) post-transcriptionally downregulates tumor suppressor Pdcd4 and stimulates invasion, intravasation and metastasis in colorectal cancer. *Oncogene,* 27. 2128-2136.

Ataya, K.M., Valeriote, F.A. & Ramahi-Ataya, A.J. (1989). Effect of cyclophosphamide on immature rat ovary. *Cancer Res.,* 49. 1660-1664.

Bal, H.S. (1984). Effect of methoxychlor on reproductive systems of the rat. *Proc. Soc. Exp. Biol. Med.,* 176. 187-196.

Bartel, D.P. (2004). MicroRNAs: genomics, biogenesis, mechanism, and function. *Cell* 116. 281-297.

Bhattacharya, P. & Keating, A.F. (2011). Involvement of Glutathione S-transferase in 7, 12-dimethylbenz[a]anthracene metabolism in the rat ovary. *Biol Reprod special edition* 67-68.

Blumenfeld, Z., Dann, E., Avivi, I., Epelbaum, R. & Rowe, J.M. (2002). Fertility after treatment for Hodgkins disease. *Ann. Oncol.,* 13. 138-147.

Borgeest, C., Miller K.P., Gupta, R., Greenfeld, C., Hruska, K.S., Hoyer, P., & Flaws, J.A. (2004). Methoxychlor-induced atresia in the mouse involves Bcl-2 family members, but not gonadotropins or estradiol. *Biol Reprod.*, 70, 1828-1835.

Borgeest, C., Symonds, D., Mayer, L.P., Hoyer, P.B. & Flaws, J.A. (2002). Methoxychlor may cause ovarian follicular atresia and proliferation of the ovarian epithelium in the mouse. *Toxicol Sci*, 68. 2, 473-8, 1096-6080.

Borman, S.M., Christian, P.J., Sipes, I.G., & Hoyer P.B. (2000). Ovotoxicity in female Fischer rats and B6 mice induced by low-dose exposure to three polycyclic aromatic hydrocarbons: comparison through calculation of an ovotoxic index. *Toxicol Appl Pharmacol*, 167. 191-198.

Brown, C., Larocca, J., Pietruska, J., Ota, M., Anderson, L., Smith, S.D., Weston, P., Rasoulpour, T. & Hixon, M.L. (2010). Subfertility caused by altered follicular development and oocyte growth in female mice lacking PKB alpha/Akt1. *Biol Reprod*, 82. 2, 246-56, 1529-7268.

Buccione, R., Schroeder, A.S. & Eppig, J.J. (1990). Interactions between somatic cells and germ cells throughout mammalian oogenesis. *Biol. Reprod.*, 43. 543-547.

Byrne, J. (1990). Fertility and pregnancy after malignancy. *Semin Perinatol.*, 14. 423-429,

Calvin, H.I., Grosshans, K., & Blake, E.J. (1986). Estimation and manipulation of glutathione levels in prepuberal mouse ovaries and ova: relevance to sperm nucleus transformation in the fertilized egg. *Gamete Res.*, 14. 265-275.

Cantley, L.C. (2002). The phosphoinositide 3-kinase pathway. *Science*, 296. 5573, 1655-7, 1095-9203.

Carabatsos, M.J., Elvin, J., Matzuk, M.M. & Albertini, D.F. (1998). Characterization of oocyte and follicle development in growth differentiation factor-9-deficient mice. *Dev Biol.* 204. 373-384.

Carletti, M.Z., Fiedler, S.D. & Christenson, L.K. (2010). MicroRNA 21 blocks apoptosis in mouse periovulatory granulosa cells. *Biol Reprod.* 83. 286-295.

Chan, J.A., Krichevsky, A.M. & Kosik, K.S. (2005). MicroRNA-21 is an antiapoptotic factor in human glioblastoma cells. Cancer Res. 65. 6029-6033.

Chapman, R.M. (1983). Gonadal injury resulting from chemotherapy. *Am. J. Ind. Med.*, 4. 149-161.

Chen, P.Y. & Meister, G. (2005). microRNA-guided posttranscriptional gene regulation. *Biol Chem.* 386. 1205-1218.

Chen, Y., Liu, W., Chao, T., Zhang, Y., Yan, X., Gong, Y., Qiang, B., Yuan, J., Sun, M. & Peng, X. (2008). MicroRNA-21 down-regulates the expression of tumor suppressor PDCD4 in human glioblastoma cell T98G. *Cancer Lett.* 272. 197-205.

Damewood, M.D. & Groschow, L.B. (1986). Prospects for fertility after chemotherapy or radiation for neoplastic disease. *Fertil. Steril.*, 45. 443-459.

Datta, S.R., Brunet, A. & Greenberg, M.E. (1999). Cellular survival: a play in three Akts. *Genes Dev*, 13. 22, 2905-27, 0890-9369.

Desmeules, P. & Devine, P.J. (2006). Characterizing the ovotoxicity of cyclophosphamide metabolites on cultured mouse ovaries. *Toxicol. Sci.*, 90. 2, 500-509.

Devine, P.J., Rajapaska, K.S. & Hoyer, P.B. (2002). In vitro ovarian tissue and organ culture: a review. *Frontiers in Bioscience*, 7, 1979-1989.

Dnistrian, A.M., Schwartz, M.K., Fracchia, A.A., Kaufman, R.J., Hakes, T.B. & Curries, V.E. (1983). Endocrine consequences of CMF adjuvant therapy in premenopausal and postmenopausal breast cancer patients. *Cancer.*, 51. 803-807.

Dou, Z., Chattopadhyay, M., Pan, J.A., Guerriero, J.L., Jiang, Y.P., Ballou, L.M., Yue, Z., Lin, R.Z. & Zong, W.X. (2010). The class IA phosphatidylinositol 3-kinase p110-beta subunit is a positive regulator of autophagy. *J Cell Biol*, 191. 4, 827-43, 1540-8140.

Eroschenko, V.P., Abuel-Atta, A.A. & Grober, M.S. (1995). Neonatal exposures to technical methoxychlor alters ovaries in adult mice. *Reprod. Toxicol.*, 9. 379-387.

Fernandez, S.M., Keating, A.F., Christian, P.J., Sen, N., Hoying, J.B., Brooks, H.L. & Hoyer, P.B. (2008). Involvement of the KIT/KITL signaling pathway in 4-vinylcyclohexene diepoxide-induced ovarian follicle loss in rats. *Biol Reprod*, 79. 2, 318-27, 0006-3363.

Foletta, V.C., Segal, D.H. & Cohen, D.R. (1998). Transcriptional regulation in the immune system: all roads lead to AP-1. *J Leukoc Biol*, 63. 2, 139-52, 0741-5400.

Frankel, L.B., Christoffersen, N.R., Jacobsen, A., Lindow, M., Krogh, A. & Lund, A.H. (2008). Programmed cell death 4 (PDCD4) is an important functional target of the microRNA miR-21 in breast cancer cells. *J Biol Chem.* 283. 1026-1033.

Gannon, A.M., Stampfli, M., & Foster, W.G. (2011). Cigarette Smoke Exposure Triggers Autophagy-Mediated Ovarian Follicle Loss in a Mouse Model. *Biology of Reproduction Special Edition*, 9.

Gawriluk, T.R., Hale, A.N., Flaws, J.A., Dillon, C.P., Green, D.R. & Rucker, E.B., 3rd. (2011). Autophagy is a cell survival program for female germ cells in the murine ovary. *Reproduction*, 141. 6, 759-65, 1741-7899.

Gaytan, M., Morales, C., Sanchez-Criado, J.E. & Gaytan, F. (2008). Immunolocalization of beclin 1, a bcl-2-binding, autophagy-related protein, in the human ovary: possible relation to life span of corpus luteum. *Cell Tissue Res*, 331. 2, 509-17, 0302-766X.

Gupta, R.K., Miller, K.P., Babus, J.K. & Flaws, J.A. (2006b). Methoxychlor inhibits growth and induces atresia of antral follicles through an oxidative stress pathway. *Toxicol. Sci.*, 93. 382-389.

Gupta, R.K., Schuh, R.A., Fiskum, G. & Flaws, J.A. (2006a). Methoxychlor causes mitochondrial dysfunction and oxidative damage in the mouse ovary. *Toxicol. Appl. Pharmacol.*, 216. 436-445.

Guthrie, H.D., Wall, R.J., Pursel, V.G., Foster-Frey, J.A., Donovan, D.M., Dawson, H.D., Welch, G.R. & Garrett, W.G. (2005). Follicular expression of a human beta-cell leukaemia/lymphoma-2 (Bcl-2) transgene does not decrease atresia or increase ovulation rate in swine. *Reprod Fertil Devel.* 17. 457-466.

Hill, C.S. & Treisman, R. (1995). Transcriptional regulation by extracellular signals: mechanisms and specificity. *Cell*, 80. 2, 199-211, 0092-8674.

Hirshfield, A.N. (1991). Development of follicles in the mammalian ovary. *Int Rev Cytol*, 124. 43-101, 0074-7696.

Horie, K., Takakura, K., Taii, S., Narimoto, K., Noda, Y., Nishikawa, S., Nakayama, H., Fujita, J. & Mori, T. (1991). The expression of c-kit protein during oogenesis and early embryonic development. *Biol Reprod*, 45. 4, 547-52, 0006-3363.

Hoyer, P.B. & Sipes, I.G. (1996). Assessment of follicle destruction in chemical-induced ovarian toxicity. *Annu Rev Pharmacol Toxicol*, 36. 307-31, 0362-1642. (

Hoyer, P.B. & Sipes, I.G. (1996). Assessment of follicle destruction in chemical-induced ovarian toxicity. *Annu. Rev. Pharmacol. Toxicol.*, 36. 307-331.

Hoyer, P.B. (2005). Impact of metals on ovarian function. Metals, Fertility and Reproductive Toxicity. 155-173, CRC Press, Boca Raton, Fl.

Hreinsson, J.G., Scott, J.E., Rasmussen, C., Swahn, M.L., Hsueh, A.J. & Hovatta, O. (2002). Growth differentiation factor-9 promotes the growth, development, and survival of human ovarian follicles in organ culture. *J Clin Endocrinol Metab.* 87. 316-321.

Hu, X., Christian, P., Sipes, I.G. & Hoyer, P.B. (2001a). Expression and redistribution of cellular Bad, Bax, and Bcl-X(L) protein is associated with VCD-induced ovotoxicity in rats. *Biol Reprod,* 65. 5, 1489-95, 0006-3363.

Hu, X., Christian, P.J., Thompson, K.E., Sipes, I.G. & Hoyer, P.B. (2001b). Apoptosis induced in rats by 4-vinylcyclohexene diepoxide is associated with activation of the caspase cascades. *Biol Reprod,* 65. 1, 87-93, 0006-3363.

Hu, X., Flaws, J.A., Sipes, I.G. & Hoyer, P.B. (2002). Activation of mitogen-activated protein kinases and AP-1 transcription factor in ovotoxicity induced by 4-vinylcyclohexene diepoxide in rats. *Biol Reprod,* 67. 3, 718-24, 0006-3363.

Huang, Y., Shen, X.J., Zou, Q., Wang, S.P., Tang, S.M. & Zhang, G.Z. (2011). Biological functions of microRNAs: a review. *J Physiol Biochem.* 67. 129-139.

Igawa, Y., Keating, A.F., Rajapaksa, K.S., Sipes, I.G. & Hoyer, P.B. (2009). Evaluation of ovotoxicity induced by 7, 12-dimethylbenz[a]anthracene and its 3,4-diol metabolite utilizing a rat in vitro ovarian culture system. *Toxicol Appl Pharmacol,* 234. 3, 361-9, 1096-0333.

International Agency for Research on Cancer (1994). 4-Vinylcyclohexene. IARC monographs on the evaluation of carcinogenic risks to humans: Some industrial chemicals. 60. 347.

Ip, Y.T. & Davis, R.J. (1998). Signal transduction by the c-Jun N-terminal kinase (JNK)-from inflammation to development. *Curr Opin Cell Biol,* 10. 2, 205-19, 0955-0674.

Ismail, R.S., Okawara, Y., Fryer, J.N. & Vanderhyden, B.C. (1996). Hormonal regulation of the ligand for c-kit in the rat ovary and its effects on spontaneous oocyte meiotic maturation. *Mol Reprod Dev,* 43. 4, 458-69, 1040-452X.

Jagarlamudi, K., Liu, L., Adhikari, D., Reddy, P., Idahl, A., Ottander, U., Lundin, E. & Liu, K. (2009). Oocyte-specific deletion of Pten in mice reveals a stage-specific function of PTEN/PI3K signaling in oocytes in controlling follicular activation. *PLoS One,* 4. 7, e6186, 1932-6203.

Jarrell, J., Lai, E.V., Barr, R., Mcmahon, A., Belbeck, L. & O'Connell, G. (1987). Ovarian toxicity of cyclophosphamide alone and in combination with ovarian irradiation in the rat. *Cancer Res.,* 47. 2340-2343.

Jick, H. & Porter, J. (1977). Relation between smoking and age of natural pregnancy. *Lancet,* 1. 1354-1355,

John, G.B., Gallardo, T.D., Shirley, L.J. & Castrillon, D.H. (2008). Foxo3 is a PI3K-dependent molecular switch controlling the initiation of oocyte growth. *Dev Biol,* 321. 1, 197-204, 1095-564X.

Johnson, N.L., Gardner, A.M., Diener, K.M., Lange-Carter, C.A., Gleavy, J., Jarpe, M.B., Minden, A., Karin, M., Zon, L.I. & Johnson, G.L. (1996). Signal transduction pathways regulated by mitogen-activated/extracellular response kinase kinase kinase induce cell death. *J Biol Chem,* 271. 6, 3229-37, 0021-9258.

Keating, A.F., C, J.M., Sen, N., Sipes, I.G. & Hoyer, P.B. (2009). Effect of phosphatidylinositol-3 kinase inhibition on ovotoxicity caused by 4-

vinylcyclohexene diepoxide and 7, 12-dimethylbenz[a]anthracene in neonatal rat ovaries. *Toxicol Appl Pharmacol*, 241. 2, 127-34, 1096-0333.

Keating, A.F., Rajapaksa, K.S., Sipes, I.G. & Hoyer, P.B. (2008a). Effect of CYP2E1 gene deletion in mice on expression of microsomal epoxide hydrolase in response to VCD exposure. *Toxicol Sci*, 105. 2, 351-9, 1096-0929.

Keating, A.F., Sen, N., Sipes, I.G. & Hoyer, P.B. (2010). Dual protective role for Glutathione S-transferase class pi against VCD-induced ovotoxicity in the rat ovary. *Toxicol Appl Pharmacol*, 1096-0333.

Keating, A.F., Sipes, I.G. & Hoyer, P.B. (2008b). Expression of ovarian microsomal epoxide hydrolase and glutathione S-transferase during onset of VCD-induced ovotoxicity in B6C3F(1) mice. *Toxicol Appl Pharmacol*, 230. 1, 109-16, 0041-008X.

Koyama, H., Wada, T., Nishizawa, Y., Iwanaga, T., Aoki, Y., Terasawa, T., Kosaki, G., Yamamoto, T. & Wada, A. (1977). Cyclophosphamide-induced ovarian failure and its therapeutic significance in patients with breast cancer. *Cancer.*, 39. 1403-1409.

Krarup, T. (1967). 9,10-Dimethyl-1,2-benzanthracene induced ovarian tumors in mice. *Acta. Pathol. Microbiol. Scand.*, 70. 241-248.

Krarup, T. (1969). Ocyte destruction and ovarian tumorigenesis after direct application of a chemical carcinogen (9,10-dimethyl-benzanthracene) to the mouse ovary. *Int. J. Cancer.*, 4. 61.

Krarup, T. (1970). Oocyte survival in the mouse ovary after treatment with 9,10-1,2-benzanthracene. *J. Endocrinol.*, 46. 483-495.

Krishna, S., Low, I.C. & Pervaiz, S. (2011). Regulation of mitochondrial metabolism: yet another facet in the biology of the oncoprotein Bcl-2. *Biochem J*, 435. 3, 545-51, 1470-8728.

Liang, X.H., Jackson, S., Seaman, M., Brown, K., Kempkes, B., Hibshoosh, H. & Levine, B. (1999). Induction of autophagy and inhibition of tumorigenesis by beclin 1. *Nature*, 402. 6762, 672-6, 0028-0836.

Liu, K., Rajareddy, S., Liu, L., Jagarlamudi, K., Boman, K., Selstam, G. & Reddy, P. (2006). Control of mammalian oocyte growth and early follicular development by the oocyte PI3 kinase pathway: new roles for an old timer. *Dev Biol*, 299. 1, 1-11, 0012-1606.

Liu, L., Rajareddy, S., Reddy, P., Du, C., Jagarlamudi, K., Shen, Y., Gunnarsson, D., Selstam, G., Boman, K. & Liu, K. (2007). Infertility caused by retardation of follicular development in mice with oocyte-specific expression of Foxo3a. *Development*, 134. 1, 199-209, 0950-1991.

Liu, L., Rajareddy, S., Reddy, P., Jagarlamudi, K., Du, C., Shen, Y., Guo, Y., Boman, K., Lundin, E., Ottander, U., Selstam, G. & Liu, K. (2007). Phosphorylation and inactivation of glycogen synthase kinase-3 by soluble kit ligand in mouse oocytes during early follicular development. *J Mol Endocrinol*, 38. 1-2, 137-46, 0952-5041.

Lopez, S.G. & Luderer, U. (2004). Effects of cyclophosphamide and buthionine sulfoximine on ovarian glutathione and apoptosis. *Free Radic Biol Med*, 36. 11, 1366-77, 0891-5849.

Luderer, U., Kavanagh, T.J., White, C.C. & Faustman, E.M. (2001). Gonadotropin regulation of glutathione synthesis in the rat ovary. *Reprod Toxicol*, 15. 5, 495-504, 0890-6238.

Manova, K., Nocka, K., Besmer, P. & Bachvarova, R.F. (1990). Gonadal expression of c-kit encoded at the W locus of the mouse. *Development*, 110. 4, 1057-69, 0950-1991.

Maronpot, R.R. (1987). Ovarian toxicity and carcinogenicity in eight recent National Toxicological Program studies. *Environ. Health Perspect.*, 73. 125-130.

Marshall, C.J. (1995). Specificity of receptor tyrosine kinase signaling: transient versus sustained extracellular signal-regulated kinase activation. *Cell*, 80. 2, 179-85, 0092-8674.

Matikainen, T., Perez, G.I., Jurisicova, A., Pru, J.K., Schlezinger, J.J., Ryu, H.Y., Laine, J., Sakai, T., Korsmeyer, S.J., Casper, R.F., Sherr, D.H. & Tilly, J.L. (2001). Aromatic hydrocarbon receptor-driven Bax gene expression is required for premature ovarian failure caused by biohazardous environmental chemicals. *Nat Genet*, 28. 4, 355-60, 1061-4036.

Mattison, D.R. & Schulman, J.D. (1980). How xenobiotic chemicals can destroy oocytes. *Contemp. Obstet. Gynecol.*, 15. 157.

Mattison, D.R. & Thorgeirsson, S.S. (1979). Ovarian aryl hydrocarbon hydroxylase activity and primordial oocyte toxicity of polycyclic aromatic hydrocarbons in mice. *Cancer Res.*, 39. 3471-3475.

Mattison, D.R., Shiromizu, K., Perndergrass, J.A. & Thoirgeirsson, S.S. (1983). Ontogeny of ovarian glutathions and sensitivity to primordial oocyte destruction by cyclophosphamide. *Pediatr. Pharmacol.*, 3. 49-55.

Melnick, R.L., Huff, J., Chou, B.J. & Miller, R.A. (1990). Carcinogenicity of 1,3-butadiene in C57BL/6 X C3HF1 mice at low exposure concentrations. *Cancer Res.*, 50. 6592-6599.

Miller, J.J.& Cole, L.J. (1970). Changes in mouse ovaries after prolonged treatment with cyclophosphamide. *Proc. Soc. Exp. biol. Med.*, 133. 190-193.

Miller, J.J., Williams, G.F. & Leissring, J.C. (1971). Multiple late complications of therapy with cyclophosphamide, including ovarian destruction. *Am. J. Med.*, 50. 530-535.

Miller, K.P., Gupta, R.K. & Flaws, J.A. (2006). Methoxychlor metabolites may cause ovarian toxicity through estrogen-regulated pathways. *Toxicol. Sci.*, 93. 180-188.

Miller, K.P., Gupta, R.K., Greenfeld, C.R., Babus, J.K. & Flaws, J.A. (2005). Methoxychlor directly affects ovarian antral follicle growth and atresia through Bcl-2- and Bax-mediated pathways. *Toxicol. Sci.*, 88. 213-221.

Morita, Y. & Tilly, J.L. (1999). Oocyte apoptosis: like sand through an hourglass. *Dev Biol*, 213. 1, 1-17, 0012-1606.

Murono, E.P & Derk, R.C. (2005). The reported active metabolite of methoxychlor, 2,2-bis(p-hydroxyphenyl)-1,1,1-trichloroethane, inhibits testosterone formation by cultured Leydig cells from neonatal rats. *Reprod. Toxicol.*, 20. 503-513.

Nilsson, E.E. & Skinner, M.K. (2002). Growth and differentiation factor-9 stimulates progression of early primary but not primordial rat ovarian follicle development. *Biol Reprod.* 67. 1018-1024.

Orr-Urtreger, A., Avivi, A., Zimmer, Y., Givol, D., Yarden, Y. & Lonai, P. (1990). Developmental expression of c-kit, a proto-oncogene encoded by the W locus. *Development*, 109. 4, 911-23, 0950-1991.

Paulini, F. & Melo, E.O. (2011). The role of oocyte-secreted factors GDF9 and BMP15 in follicular development and oogenesis. *Reprod Dom Anim.* 46. 354-361.

Pawson, T. & Nash, P. (2000). Protein-protein interactions define specificity in signal transduction. *Genes Dev*, 14. 9, 1027-47, 0890-9369.

Pendergast, A.M. (2002) The Abl family kinases: mechanisms of regulation and signaling. *Adv Cancer Res.* 85. 51-100.

Plowchalk, D.R. & Mattison, D.R. (1992). Reproductive toxicity of cyclophosphamide in the C57GBL/6N mouse. 1. Effects on ovarian structure and function. *Reprod. Toxicol.*, 6. 411-421.

Pru, J.K., Kaneko-Tarui, T., Jurisicova, A., Kashiwagi, A., Selesniemi, K. & Tilly, J.L. (2009). Induction of proapoptotic gene expression and recruitment of p53 herald ovarian follicle loss caused by polycyclic aromatic hydrocarbons. *Reprod Sci*, 16. 4, 347-56, 1933-7205.

Rajapaksa, K.S., Cannady, E.A., Sipes, I.G. & Hoyer, P.B. (2007). Involvement of CYP 2E1 enzyme in ovotoxicity caused by 4-vinylcyclohexene and its metabolites. *Toxicol Appl Pharmacol*, 221. 2, 215-21, 0041-008X.

Rajapaksa, K.S., Sipes, I.G. & Hoyer, P.B. (2007). involvement of microsomal epoxide hydrolase enzyme in ovotoxicity caused by 7,12-dimethylbenz[a]anthracene. *Toxicol Sci*, 96. 2, 327-34, 1096-6080.

Rajareddy, S., Reddy, P., Du, C., Liu, L., Jagarlamudi, K., Tang, W., Shen, Y., Berthet, C., Peng, S.L., Kaldis, P. & Liu, K. (2007). p27kip1 (cyclin-dependent kinase inhibitor 1B) controls ovarian development by suppressing follicle endowment and activation and promoting follicle atresia in mice. *Mol Endocrinol*, 21. 9, 2189-202, 0888-8809.

Reddy, P., Adhikari, D., Zheng, W., Liang, S., Hamalainen, T., Tohonen, V., Ogawa, W., Noda, T., Volarevic, S., Huhtaniemi, I. & Liu, K. (2009). PDK1 signaling in oocytes controls reproductive aging and lifespan by manipulating the survival of primordial follicles. *Hum Mol Genet*, 18. 15, 2813-24, 1460-2083.

Reddy, P., Liu, L., Adhikari, D., Jagarlamudi, K., Rajareddy, S., Shen, Y., Du, C., Tang, W., Hamalainen, T., Peng, S.L., Lan, Z.J., Cooney, A.J., Huhtaniemi, I. & Liu, K. (2008). Oocyte-specific deletion of Pten causes premature activation of the primordial follicle pool. *Science*, 319. 5863, 611-3, 1095-9203.

Reddy, P., Shen, L., Ren, C., Boman, K., Lundin, E., Ottander, U., Lindgren, P., Liu, Y.X., Sun, Q.Y. & Liu, K. (2005). Activation of Akt (PKB) and suppression of FKHRL1 in mouse and rat oocytes by stem cell factor during follicular activation and development. *Dev Biol*, 281. 2, 160-70, 0012-1606.

Reddy, P., Zheng, W. & Liu, K. (2010). Mechanisms maintaining the dormancy and survival of mammalian primordial follicles. *Trends Endocrinol Metab*, 21. 2, 96-103, 1879-3061.

Richards, J.S. (1980). Maturation of ovarian follicles: actions and interactions of pituitary and ovarian hormones on follicular cell differentiation. *Physiol. Rev*, 60. 51-89.

Rincon, M., Whitmarsh, A., Yang, D.D., Weiss, L., Derijard, B., Jayaraj, P., Davis, R.J. & Flavell, R.A. (1998). The JNK pathway regulates the in vivo deletion of immature CD4(+)CD8(+) thymocytes. *J Exp Med*, 188. 10, 1817-30, 0022-1007.

Roskoski, R., Jr. (2005a). Signaling by Kit protein-tyrosine kinase--the stem cell factor receptor. *Biochem Biophys Res Commun*, 337. 1, 1-13, 0006-291X.

Roskoski, R., Jr. (2005b). Structure and regulation of Kit protein-tyrosine kinase--the stem cell factor receptor. *Biochem Biophys Res Commun*, 338. 3, 1307-15, 0006-291X.

She, Q.B., Solit, D.B., Ye, Q., O'reilly, K.E., Lobo, J. & Rosen, N. (2005). The BAD protein integrates survival signaling by EGFR/MAPK and PI3K/Akt kinase pathways in PTEN-deficient tumor cells. *Cancer Cell*, 8, 287-297.

Sobinoff, A.P., Mahony, M., Nixon, B., Roman, S.D. & McLaughlin, E.A. (2011). Understanding the villian: DMBA induced pre-antral ovotoxicity involves selective follicular destruction and primordial follicle activation through PI3K/Akt and mTOR signaling. *Toxicol. Sci. In press.*

Sobrinho, L.G., Levine, R.A. & Deconti, R.C. (1971). Amenhorrhea in patients with Hodkins disease treated wth antineoplastic agents. *Am. J. Obstet. Gynecol.*, 109. 135-139.

Springer, L.N., Flaws, J.A., Sipes, I.G. & Hoyer, P.B. (1996). Follicular mechanisms associated with 4-vinylcyclohexene diepoxide-induced ovotoxicity in rats. *Reprod Toxicol*, 10. 2, 137-43, 0890-6238.

Symonds, D.A., Merchenthaler, I. & Flaws, J.A. (2009). Methoxychlor and estradiol induce oxidative stress DNA damage in the mouse ovarian surface epithelium. *Toxicol Sci.*, 105. 182-187.

Tilly, J.L., Kowalski, K.I., Johnson, A.L. & Hsueh, A.J. (1991). Involvement of apoptosis in ovarian follicular atresia and postovulatory regression. *Endocrinol.*, 129. 2799.

Tingen, C.M., Bristol-Gould, S.K., Kiesewetter, S.E., Wellington, J.T., Shea, L. & Woodruff, T.K. (2009). Prepubertal primordial follicle loss in mice is not due to classical apoptotic pathways. *Biol Reprod*, 81. 1, 16-25, 0006-3363.

Tomic, D., Frech, M.S., Babus, J.K., Gupta, R.K., Furth, P.A., Koos, R.D. & Flaws, J.A. (2006). Methoxychlor induces atresia of antral follicles in ERalpha-overexpressing mice. *Toxicol. Sci.*, 93. 196-204.

Tsai-Turton, M., Nakamura, B.N. & Luderer, U. (2007). Induction of apoptosis by 9,10-dimethyl-1,2-benzanthracene in cultured preovulatory rat follicles is preceded by a rise in reactive oxygen species and is prevented by glutathione. *Biol Reprod*, 77. 3, 442-51, 0006-3363.

Tsujimoto, Y. & Shimizu, S. (2005). Another way to die: autophagic programmed cell death. *Cell Death Differ.* 12. 1528-1534.

Vahakangas, K., Rajaniemi, H. & Pelkonen, O. (1985). Ovarian toxicity of cigarette smoke during pregnancy in mice. *Toxicol Lett*, 25. 75.

Warne, G.L., Fairley, K.F., Hobbs, J.B. & Martin, F.I.R. (1973). Cyclophosphamide-induced ovarian failure. *N. Engl. J. Med.*, 289. 1159-1162.

Whitmarsh, A.J. & Davis, R.J. (1996). Transcription factor AP-1 regulation by mitogen-activated protein kinase signal transduction pathways. *J Mol Med (Berl)*, 74. 10, 589-607, 0946-2716.

Whitworth, K.M., Agca, C., Kim, J.G., Patel, R.V., Springer, G.K., Bivens, N.J., Forrester, L.J., Mathialagan, N., Green, J.A. & Prather, R.S. (2005). Transcriptional profiling of pig embryogenesis by using a 15-K member unigene set specific for pig reproductive tissues and embryos. *Biol Reprod.* 72. 1437-1451.

Xia, Z., Dickens, M., Raingeaud, J., Davis, R.J. & Greenberg, M.E. (1995). Opposing effects of ERK and JNK-p38 MAP kinases on apoptosis. *Science*, 270. 5240, 1326-31, 0036-8075.

Yang, M.Y. & Rajamahendran, R. (2002). Expression of Bcl-2 and Bax proteins in relation to quality of bovine oocytes and embryos produced in vitro. *Anim Reprod Sci.* 70. 159-169.

Yoon, S.J., Kim, E.Y., Kim, Y.S., Lee, H.S., Kim, K.H., Bae, J. & Lee, K.A. (2009). Role of Bcl2-like 10 (Bcl2l10) in Regulating Mouse Oocyte Maturation. *Biol Reprod.* 81. 497-506.

Zanke, B.W., Boudreau, K., Rubie, E., Winnett, E., Tibbles, L.A., Zon, L., Kyriakis, J., Liu, F.F. & Woodgett, J.R. (1996). The stress-activated protein kinase pathway mediates cell death following injury induced by cis-platinum, UV irradiation or heat. *Curr Biol*, 6. 5, 606-13, 0960-9822.

Zhu, S., Si, M.L., Wu, H. & Mo, Y.Y. (2007). MicroRNA-21 targets the tumor suppressor gene tropomyosin 1 (TPM1). *J Biol Chem*. 282. 14328-14336.

Zhu, S., Wu, H., Wu, F., Nie, D., Sheng, S. & Mo, Y.Y. (2008). MicroRNA-21 targets tumor suppressor genes in invasion and metastasis. *Cell Res*. 18. 350-359.

4

Fertility Preservation in Gynecologic Cancers Patients

Valeria I. Farfalli and Hector D. Ferreyra
National University of Cordoba,
Argentina

1. Introduction

Infertility can arise as a consequence of treatment of oncological conditions. (5) The parallel and continued improvement in both, the management of oncology and fertility cases in recent times, has brought to the fore-front the potential for fertility preservation in patients being treated for cancer. (26)(27)

Clearly Oncologists must be aware of situations where their treatment wills affect fertility in patients who are being treated for cancer and they must also be aware of the pathways available for procedures such as cryopreservation of gametes and/or embryos. (6)

This surge in activity is based largely on the improved survival of women and girls from malignant disease. This has been particularly so in paediatric oncology, with a transformation from very low success rates for many conditions to the current situation where 80-90% of children with cancer can expect to survive long term. (1)

The loss of fertility is a common consequence of the use of many therapeutic agents for non-malignant as well as malignant conditions, including systemic lupus erythematosis and other rheumatological diseases. Bone marrow stem cell transplantation with chemotherapy conditioning is now being used in many other conditions.

Some people are at risk for impaired fertility or infertility because of exposure to occupational or environmental hazards and thus might want to take measures to preserve their fertility. For example, some industries, particularly textiles, clinical laboratories, manufacturing, printing, and dry cleaning, frequently involve exposure to chemical hazards. Health-care workers can receive significant exposures to gonadotoxic agents such as estrogenic compounds, anesthetic gases, and chemotherapeutics, or compounds that can exert embryotoxic, teratogenic, or carcinogenic effects on the zygote, embryo, or fetus. Exposure to biologic agents (e.g., cytomegalovirus, hepatitis B virus, human immunodeficiency virus, human parvovirus B19, Listeria monocytogenes, rubella virus, or varicella/herpes zoster virus) also exposes risks to reproductive health. Also military personnel might want to take measures to preserve their fertility due to a risk of exposure to radiation, biologic, or chemical agents that can compromise their fertility. Furthermore, some individuals live in communities that could disproportionately expose them to pesticides, lead, and other toxins.

Female cancer patients between the ages of fifteen and forty-nine years are expected to not only survive their disease but also lead normal lives, mainly because of newer, more effective cancer therapies such as sterilizing chemotherapy and/or radiotherapy. (3) Consequently, fertility preservation has become an important quality-of-life issue. Problems with fertility and obstetric disorders such as early pregnancy loss, premature labor, and low birth weight have all been described after cancer treatment. (1)

There is a range of alternative options to preserve fertility, based on the type and timing of chemotherapy, the type of cancer, the patient's age and the partner status.

Fertility preservation should be an integral part of improving the quality of life in cancer survivors. However it is neither possible nor ethical to recommend the same recipe for every cancer patient.

2. The impact of oncology therapy on fertility

2.1 Surgical management

Surgery can impact on fertility. It can either render someone infertile by removal of reproductive organs or it can be affected by complications of surgery. There is no doubt, however, that in recent years there has been a tendency towards more conservative treatment for many malignancies affecting the reproductive organs.(16)

In women, there has been tendency towards less radical approaches to **cervical cancer** with the development of loop excision techniques for premalignant cervix lesions or in situ carcinoma and more recently the development of the radical abdominal and vaginal trachelectomy indicated in cervical cancer lesions stage I less than 2 cm (fig. 1), which allows a radical approach to cervix cancer that is treatable surgically, but with preservation of the uterus and thus fertility. (28)(22)

Endometrial cancer is usually a disease of the postmenopausal group or at least in those who have had completed their family, and therefore it's unusual for treatment of this disease, which does involve hysterectomy and bilateral oophorectomy, to impact upon fertility. Today exist the possibility to detect early stage well-differentiated tumors that can be treated with resection of the lesion and progestin therapy. (29)

Epithelial **ovarian cancer** continues to be treated radically with loss of reproductive organs. But increasing understanding of germ cell malignancies, borderline tumours of the ovary and epithelial tumors at stage IA grade I, has led to a more conservative approach to these neoplasms and often a single oophorectomy will be performed where in the past, a hysterectomy and/or bilateral oophorectomy would have been the treatment of choice. (10)

It is unusual for **vulvar carcinoma** to be seen in the reproductive age group, and although it may have major psychosexual impact is unusual that surgical treatment impact upon fertility. In the case of early-stage vulvar cancer, the radical excision of the lesion and removing and examining one or two sentinel nodes in the groin and upper leg is an effective way to detect whether cancer has spread, but also results in fewer adverse side effects with great results and without being a posible cause of infertility. (10)

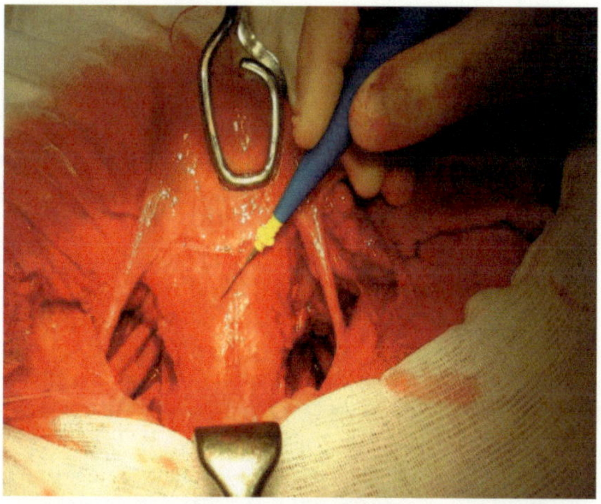

A.

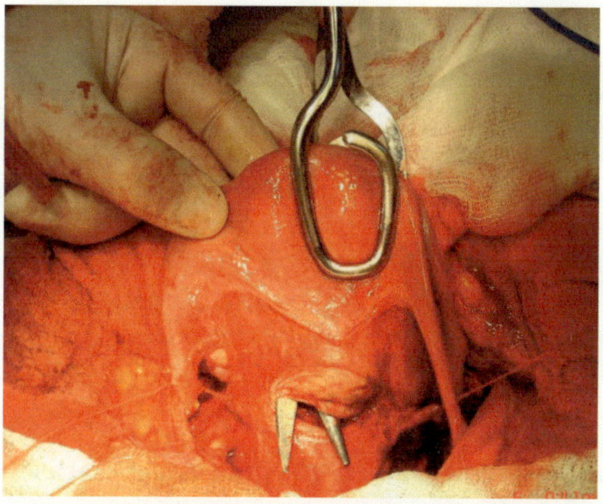

B.

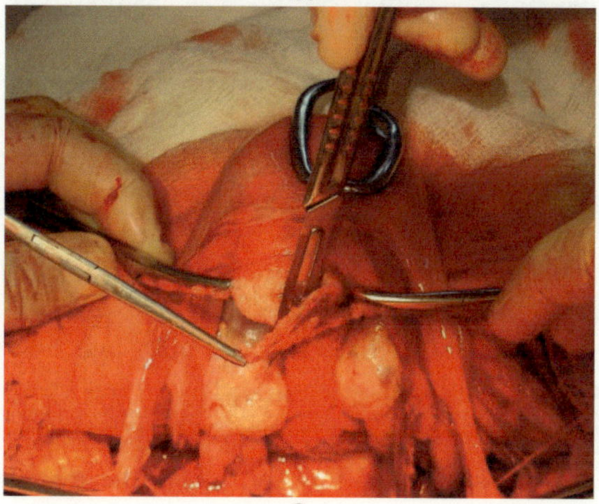

C.

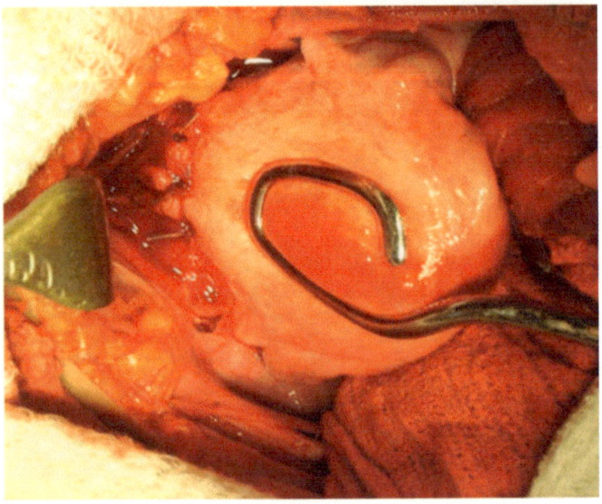

D.

Fig. 1. Radical Abdominal Trachelectomy for cancer of the cervix. A-B-C-D surgery stages.

2.2 Effects of chemotherapy and radiotherapy

With the improved survival rate of childhood and young adult cancer patients, the long-term sequelae of the treatments used are increasingly important. Current knowledge of the gonadotoxicity of commonly employed chemotherapeutic agents and radiotherapy regimens is needed to differenciate between the effect of "high-risk" and "low-risk" agents tailoring treatment to suit the individual and counseling patients regarding reduced fertility have resulted in the best practice.

2.2.1 Chemotherapy

Chemotherapy can produce significant effects upon patient fertility. (27)(26) These effects are dependent on a number of factors:

- Radical versus adjuvant chemotherapy. Radical chemotherapy generally has more profound effects on fertility than adjuvant chemotherapy,
- Single agent versus combination chemotherapy. Increasing complexities of regimes are more likely to have impacts upon fertility than single agent,
- Dose-dependent effects. Increasing doses are likely to have more profound effects on fertility than lower doses,
- Drug-dependent effects. Different agents have a markedly different impact upon fertility with some chemo-therapeutic agents sparing fertility while others are extremely toxic in this regard,
- Age-dependent effects. In the female in particular, age has a profound effect on chemotherapy toxicity.

Chemotherapy regimens administered to women under the age of 40 have a much higher chance of regaining the normal ovarian function whilst the majority of women over 40, administered toxic chemotherapy will be rendered menopausal by their treatment.

Presumably part of the reason for this is the fact that the natural attrition rate of oocyte sees a large drop in oocyte numbers over age 40 (decreased ovarian reserve) and this corresponds with decreased live birth rates in fertility patients over the age of 40.

Detailed information regarding fertility effects of many chemotherapy regimes is lacking, but specific examples where chemotherapy affects fertility is documented include the following.

Toxic effects of commonly used chemotherapeutic agents

A fixed number of primordial follicles present at birth form the ovarian reserve into puberty. Postpuberty these primordial follicles contain single oocytes arrested in the prophase of the first meiotic division and are highly sensitive to cytotoxic drugs leading to cellular death.

Follicular depletion has been shown to be physiologically age dependent, the maximum rate of depletion occurring around the age of 38 years when the reserve is just about 10% the number present at menarche. The gonadal toxic effect is thus not just dependent on type(s) and dosage of the cytotoxic drug(s) employed but also on the age of the woman.

Cell cycle nonspecific agents such as cyclophosphamide (alkylating agent) are very gonadotoxic because they destroy resting primordial cells as opposed to cell cycle specific agents such as methotrexate (antimetabolite) and Antibiotics which spare the rest primordial cells and, as such, are less gonadotoxic.

The toxicity of chemotherapy on the ovary depends on the type of drug, the mechanism of action and the age of the patient. Alkylating agents are among the most gonadotoxic, and cyclophosphamide remain the most important since it is widely used in therapeutic regimens, especially for breast cancer. The dose of cyclophosphamide that leads to ovarian failure is age dependent, since for example requires 20.4 g for a patient aged 20 to 29 years to start with amenorrhea while for a patient over 40 years only takes 5.5 grams of cumulative dose to a total ovarian failure. Moreover, there are drugs with minimal gonadotoxic effects as antimetabolites (methotrexate and fluorouracil), alkaloids (vincristine or etopocide) and antibiotics (actinomycin-D, doxorubicin and bleomycin). The patients treated for gestational throfoblastic disease and ovarian tumors of germ line, that use this type of drugs have low gonatotoxic effect preserving the possibility of future fertility.

So we can conclude based on what we observed that:

i. Adriamycin and cyclophosphamide have a 38% ovarian failure rate in women aged over 40 years at 2 years post chemotherapy.
ii. Cyclophosphamide, Hydroxydaunorubicin (Adriamycin) Oncovin (vincristine), and Prednisolone do not usually lead to permanent amenorrhoea in women under 40 years of age, but may lead to early menopause in older women.
iii. ABVD (Doxorubicin, Bleomycin, Vinblastin, and Dacarbazine) used in the treatment of Hodgkin's disease is significantly less toxic in terms of fertility than the older MOPP (Mechlorethamine, Vincristine, Procarbazine and Prednisolone).
iv. Bleomycin and doxorubicin have minimal effects on fertility.
v. Vinca alkaloids and antimetabolites have very mild effects on fertility (Methotrexate very mild at 6 gm total dose).

vi. Taxanes are not clearly defined in terms of their impact on fertility.
vii. Cyclophosphamide, methotrexate, and 5-fluorouracil (CMF) a classical breast cancer regime will render 71% of women over 40 years of age amenorrhoeic at 2 years.(25)(24)

2.2.2 Radiotherapy

The principle of radiotherapy is based on the ionisation of cellular atoms and molecules leading to the destruction of double and single DNA structures within the cell structure.

A chain of events is set up, disrupting the cell-cycle leading to apoptosis of the cells. Radiotherapy has its use in oncology because unlike malignant cells, most normal cells have the inert ability to recover from the effects of radiotherapy.

Clearly radiotherapy can be administered as external beam therapy (teletherapy), or as intracavity (brachytherapy) treatments. In addition to this, radiotherapy can be given with radical curative intent or as adjuvant therapy often postoperatively.

The direct effects of radiotherapy are dose dependent and are also dependent on the field applied to the individual. It is important to consider the effect of scattered radiation as well as direct irradiation when assessing likely effects on fertility. (25)

The application of 14.3 Gray to an ovary in a woman over 30 years of age will usually render her irreversibly infertile and menopausal. A dose of 6 Gray to the ovary of a woman less than 30 years of age is usually reversible, but ultimately, will bring the menopause forwards.

Thus the female is not only concerned with issues regarding fertility but also with hormone production, as both seem to be equally affected by radiotherapy.

Although the uterus is relatively resistant to radiotherapy there is no doubt that uterine irradiation is harmful and even if fertility is conserved, uterine irradiation will result in poor implantation. This appears to be due to a number of factors including reduced uterine volume and blood flow which have been demonstrated to result in increased mid-trimester losses, preterm labour and intrauterine growth retardation. (1)

The vagina is relatively radio-resistant however; irradiation of this organ carries with it the risk of loss of lubrication and stenosis which may result in physical impairments to fertility as well as major psychosexual issues. (1)

3. Options for fertility preservation

As illustrated in Figure 2, there is a range of clinical scenarios in which different fertility preservation techniques are appropriate. These can be discussed with the patient or, in the case of a child, with the patient and her parents. (8)

The American Society of Clinical Oncology (ASCO), the American Society for Reproductive Medicine and the NICE guidance recommend that all such patients of childbearing age be informed about fertility preservation treatment options. Despite these recommendations and the expanding availability of fertility preservation services, surveys of oncologists have revealed that only a small minority of eligible patients are referred to reproductive endocrinologist for fertility preservation counselling. (17)(18)

Current fertility preservation treatment options include emergency embryo an oocyte cryopreservation and ovarian tissue freezing.

The most successful alternative for female survivors is embryo cryopreservation, which is available in all IVF units (In Vitro Fertilization), an approach not suitable for many single women or even possible for prepuberal girls.

Preserving fertility through the cryopreservation of ovarian tissues or oocytes (although still in experimental stages) would increase the chances that children or single women could someday become parents even after exposure to chemotherapy or other agents that can cause infertility. (9)(11)

When there is ovarian involvement, or when potential for occult metastasis is high, however, ovarian tissue should not be cryopreserved for the purpose of autotransplantation. In theory, normal appearing ovarian tissue can be cryopreserved with the idea of future in vitro maturation of primordial follicles and xenografting. (12)

Preventing reproductive failure would be an ideal approach. Research is under way to evaluate treatment with gonadotropin-realising hormones (GnRh) in conjunction with chemotherapy, inducing a transient prepubertal state that might reduce the damage to reproductive organs and thereby prevent oocyte death during cancer treatment.

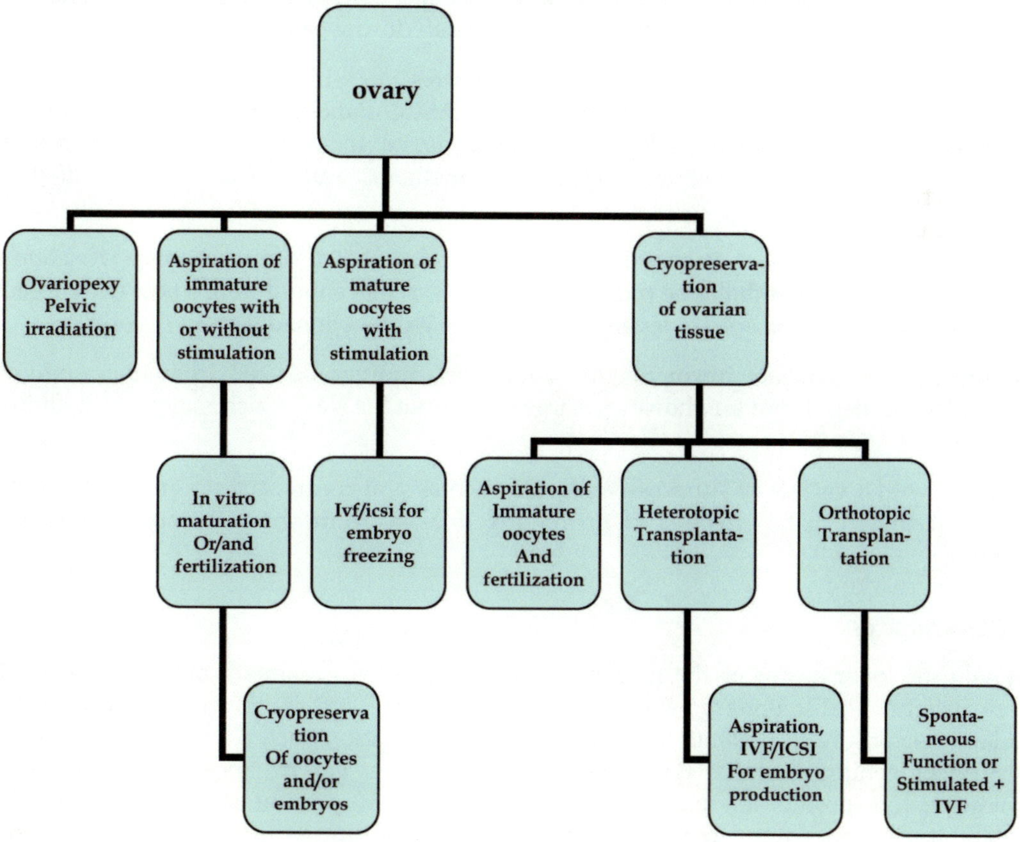

Fig. 2. Fertility Preservation options.

However, fertility preservation using ovarian suppression with GnRh agonists should still be considered experimental. In fact, members of ASCO Panel recommend that interested patients enrol onto clinical trials specifically designed to evaluate the effectiveness of fertility preservation by ovarian suppression methods, rather than receive off-study treatment.

Other strategies under development include producing oocytes from stem cells and regenerating oocytes by inducing natural mechanisms.

It is a central dogma of female reproductive biology that oogenesis ceases around the time of birth in mammalian species. In 2004, one study published by Johnson et al. (30), in which they claimed that in the adult mouse ovary, neo-oogenesis takes place and originates from female germline stem cells that are present in either the ovarian surface epithelium or bone marrow. Following these publications, experiments showed that non-germinal stem cells could generate oocytes. So at this moment there is a lot scientist trying to find the way to achieve oogenesis in adult mammals, but they are all experimental.

3.1 Chemoprotection

Preventing reproductive failure would be an ideal approach. Research is under way to evaluate treatment with gonadotropin-realising hormones (GnRh) in conjunction with chemotherapy, inducing a transient prepubertal state that might reduce the damage to reproductive organs and thereby prevent oocyte death during cancer treatment.

However, fertility preservation using ovarian suppression with GnRh agonists should still be considered experimental. In fact, members of ASCO Panel recommend that interested patients enrol onto clinical trials specifically designed to evaluate the effectiveness of fertility preservation by ovarian suppression methods, rather than receive off-study treatment.

Criticism of this approach is also derived from the fact that if the mechanism of action is primarily through hypothalamic pituitary suppression, this should not protect early follicle damage that is gonadotropin independent. However a direct gonadal effect is possible.

At present, the data are unconvincing, with most findings derived from non-randomly controlled studies. There are, however, large studies under way which may yield definitive answers.

Therapy with a variety of suppressive agents such as oral contraceptives or progestins has not been shown to be effective in preventing damage from chemotherapy or radiation therapy.

3.2 Ovariopexy

Moving the ovaries out of the field of irradiation can help maintain ovarian function in patients scheduled to undergo gonadotoxic radiotherapy. This significantly reduces ovarian radiation exposure in patients who receive pelvic irradiation such as those with Hodkin's disease or genitourinary or low intestinal malignancies. For instance, the ovarian dose following transposition is reduced to approximately 5-10 percent of the in situ ovaries. Lateral transposition appears to be more effective than suturing the ovaries to the posterior face of the uterus.

The transposition is typically performed by laparotomy. This approach is used at the time of radical hysterectomy for cervical cancer. If there is no need of laparotomy for cancer excision, ovarian transposition should be performed laparoscopically just prior initiation of radiation therapy.

3.3 Assisted reproductive technologies

Assisted reproductive technology is probably the most used modality in patients that wish to proceed to fertility preservation. The American Society of Reproductive Medicine recognizes that there is sufficient evidence to recommend embryo cryopreservation as a routine clinical care compared with other therapeutic strategies.

3.3.1 Oocyte cryopreservation

Oocyte cryopreservation is an alternative to embryo storage and is ideal for women who do not have a partner and do not want to use donor sperm. For this procedure, the patient has to undergo ovarian stimulation and egg retrieval, the same process required for embryo cryopreservation. Oocyte cryopreservation does not require IVF or ICSI (IntraCitomasplatic Sperm Inyection), and creation of unnecessary embryos can be prevented.

Although oocyte cryopreservation is still considered experimental in the United States, this technology has proven successful. Indeed, current live-birth rates from series of frozen-thawed oocytes are comparable to those in frozen-thawed embryo cycles, and there was no apparent increase in the rate of congenital anomalies as compared with U.S. national statistics for natural conceptions as reported by the Centres for Disease Control.

Actually there are two kind of techniques used for cryopreservation of oocytes: Vitrification and slow freezing.

To date, there is no standard protocol for vitrification of oocytes, which makes an analysis of published data difficult.

Since 2005, the pregnancy rates and live-birth rates have been significantly increased in both slow freezing and vitrification groups. (19).

When the data from 1998–2008 is analyzed, oocyte survival rate was higher in the vitrified group (81%) compared with in the slow frozen group (68%). The live-birth rate per ET was 14%and 34%in the slow frozen and vitrified group, respectively.

Cryopreservation of immature oocytes at the stage of germinal vesicle (GV) can be an attractive alternative to cryopreservation of mature oocytes, especially in breast cancer patients (Figure 3). In theory, there are several advantages of GV stage oocyte cryopreservation. First of all, it does not require full ovarian stimulation, which can be a significant benefit for breast cancer patients who cannot delay cancer treatment or who have ERþ (estrogen-progestin receptors) tumor. It wills also benefit women who are at high risk for ovarian hyperstimulation syndrome such as patients with polycystic ovarian syndrome. (4)

To date, cryopreservation of immature oocytes at the GV stage has not been very successful. Nevertheless, immature oocyte cryopreservation followed by in vitro maturation can be a powerful tool for fertility preservation in breast cancer patients.

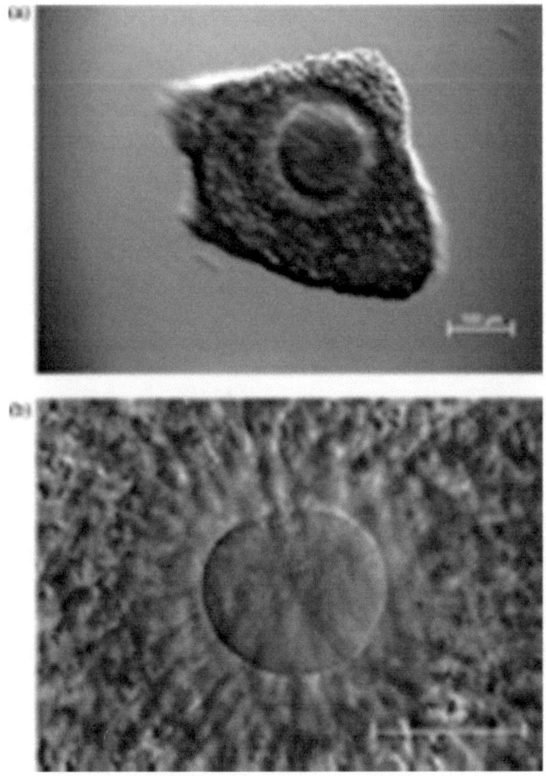

Fig. 3. Examples of GV state above and mature oocyte below.

3.3.2 Embryo cryopreservation

Embryo storage is ideal for an adult woman in a stable relationship as it is an established technique which has been available since the mid 1980s.

IVF and ICSI offer a success rate of approximately 30% per cycle (dependent on age) and this is similar to the natural conception rate that is achievable by healthy couples without assisted reproductive techniques. It involves stimulating the ovaries using gonadotrophins which results in high oestrogen levels, and certainly this raises concerns for some tumours such as breast cancers with oestrogen receptor positivity. It is still unclear what are the risks of such techniques in terms of tumour progression or relapse in a hormone dependent cancer. Some groups have attempted to address this by using tamoxifen or letrozole alone or in combination with standard IVF stimulation for women with breast cancer or endometrial cancer.

Patient numbers are small and long-term studies are currently not available. There are also no data on the pregnancy outcome from embryos generated from these protocols. However, many women and their physicians will choose not to expose an estrogen-responsive cancer to more estrogenic stimulation than is strictly necessary. (4)

IVF protocols are well defined, although it may be helpful under some circumstances to induce luteolysis with a GnRH antagonist to allow FSH injections to start sooner. GnRH antagonists also allow for a shorter duration of treatment.

IVF stimulation takes a minimum of two to three weeks depending on a patient's menstrual cycle and could be anything up to five weeks. After stimulation of follicles to maturation an egg collection procedure is undertaken usually as a day case under sedation or a general anaesthetic where vaginal ultrasound probe is used to guide transvaginal collection of eggs. IVF is then undertaken to fertilise the patient's eggs with the partner's sperm before freezing the embryo. At present there is limited availability donor sperm for adult women trying to preserve reproductive potential whilst undertaking chemotherapy (Figure 4).

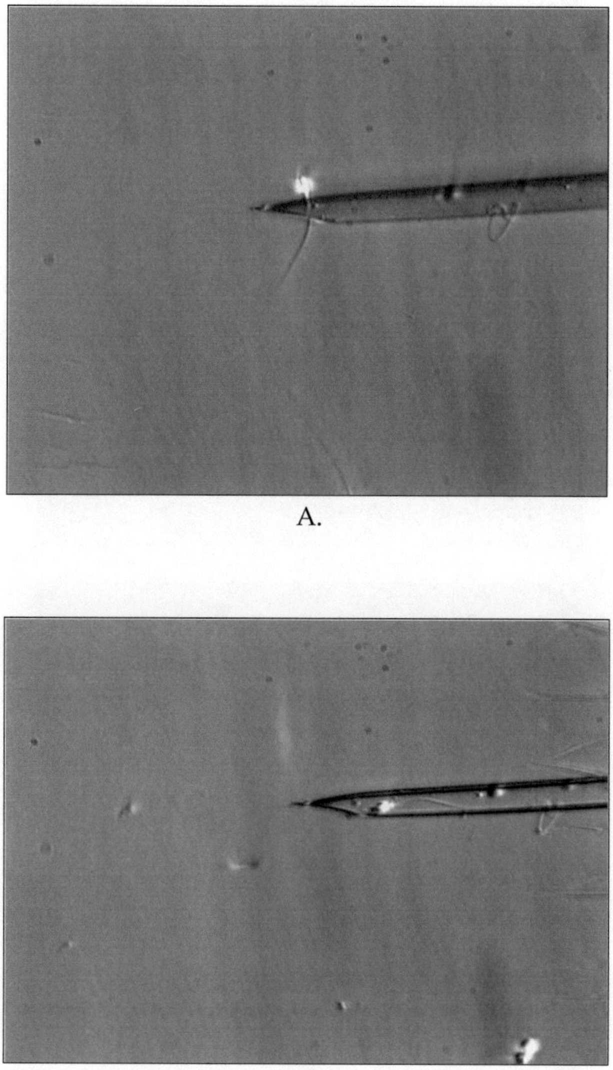

A.

B.

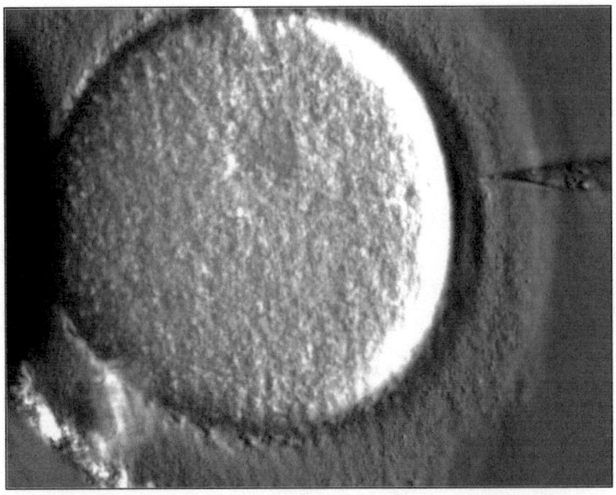

C.

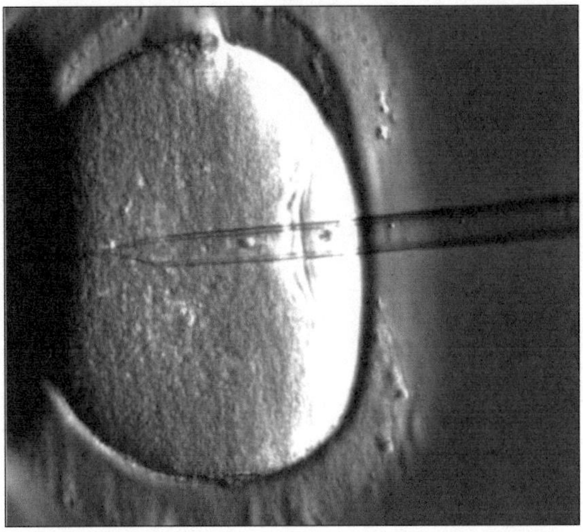

D.

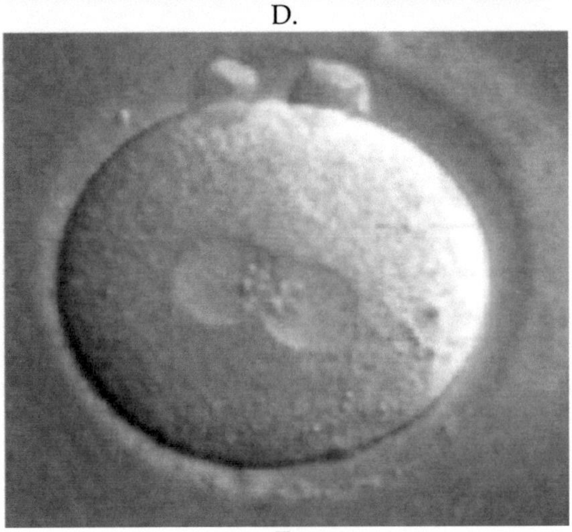

E.

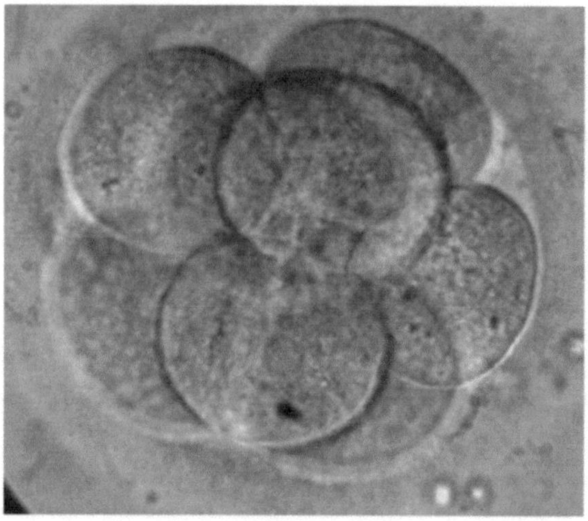

F.

A. Sperm selection for insemination into oocyte (ICSI technique)
B. Sperm aspiration.
C. Oocyte punction.
D. Introducing the sperm into the oocyte cytoplasm.
E. Fertilize oocyte at 2 pronuclear stage.
F. Embryo at 72 hs after fertilization at 8 cells stage.

Fig. 4. ICSI technique.

3.3.3 Ovarian tissue cryopreservation

An alternative option therefore is to store ovarian tissue, which may contain many more oocytes. Advantages include the fact that no other treatment is required and it can be carried out at short notice. It requires no male involvement, but does require a surgical procedure both to recover the tissue and replace it at a later date.

Replacement provides the option of spontaneous rather than assisted conception as well as the chance of more than one pregnancy; this has now been demonstrated.(11)(13)

Importantly, ovarian tissue cryopreservation also offers a potential option for children and adolescents for whom ovarian stimulation is inappropriate. This, however, may be better described as a theoretical option; as yet no adolescent girl has gone on to have a child following this procedure.

One important consideration is that a significant amount of ovarian tissue must be removed from the patient and will not therefore be available for spontaneous fertility should she not be sterilised by her cancer treatment.

At present there is debate over whether unilateral oophorectomy or ovarian biopsy is the more appropriate surgical technique.

All human trials of cryopreserved autotransplanted tissue have been with cortical strips. This concept was developed from previous work in animal models that have used cryopreserved thawed ovarian cortical strips and reported follicular survival and endocrine function as well as restoration of fertility after transplantation of cryopreserved-thawed ovarian cortical strips. Using present techniques, ovarian tissue strips are removed from the patient prior to chemotherapy. They are frozen in small strips (Figure 5). When the patient is ready for pregnancy, they are transplanted back into the patient in a heterotopic or orthotopic site. Since this is an avascular graft, up to two-thirds of follicles are lost after transplantation. Given this limitation it has been recommended that ovarian tissue freezing should be restricted to patients younger than thirty five years.

At present a total of 14 children have been born to women who have had ovarian tissue cryopreserved and reimplanted. Both spontaneous and assisted conceptions have been demonstrated, but interestingly no successful pregnancies have yet been described following heterotopic transplantation of the ovary. Sites where follicular growth has been observed include the anterior abdominal wall and the arm, although successful non-human primate pregnancies have been reported following fresh transplantation to a subcutaneous site. These approaches do, however, offer the opportunity for our improved understanding of the extra-ovarian requirements for normal follicular and oocyte development.

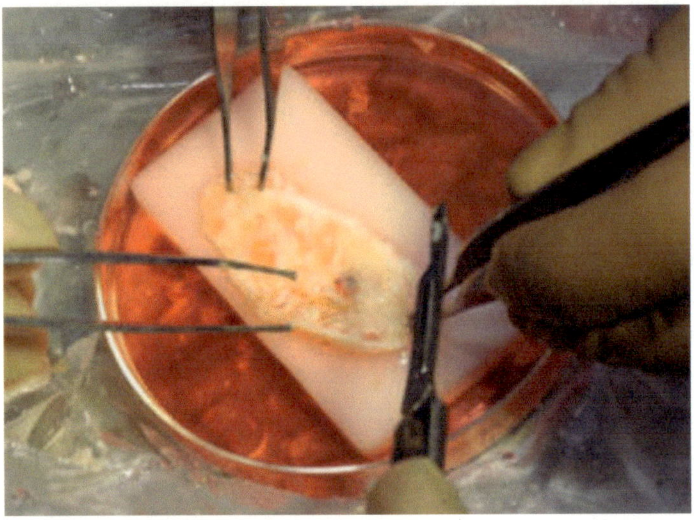

Fig. 5. Ovarian tissue preparation for cryopreservation.

The malignant contamination of the ovarian tissue must also be considered. So far, a total of some 30 women have received transplantation of ovarian tissue without any reports of relapse caused by the transplantation. Two large series of ovarian biopsies in breast cancer patients have recently revealed no evidence of malignant cell contamination, but the availability of specific molecular tumour markers in some conditions has revealed the potential for contamination. This is a particular issue for haematological malignancies; importantly, chemotherapy prior to ovarian cryopreservation did not preclude contamination. (12)

There are several potential uses of cryopreserved ovarian tissue: transplantation back into the host, in vitro maduration of primordial follicles, and xenografting into a host animal. The tissue can be transplanted back into patient.

Research should focus on refining the cryopreservation protocols, cryoprotectants, and transplantation techniques that decrease ischemia, particularly the use of vascularised grafts.

4. Facilitating fertility preservation consultation

Treating physicians should initiate the discussion of the possible treatment-related effects to fertility and indicate that there are options to safeguard their future fertility potential. (20)

Women of reproductive potential and interested in learning about options for fertility preservation should be referred real time to a reproductive endocrinologist. Preferably, a fertility preservation consultation should be arranged at the time of the initial diagnosis to expedite necessary options including COS and oocyte retrieval for embryo cryopreservation or alternative fertility preservation techniques. Using these referral mechanisms can eliminate time delays for appointments, initiate education on the process to the patient, and provide documentation such as pathology reports or treatment plans to the referring clinician. Without the development of such a streamlined process, patients and providers will experience frustration and unnecessary time delays. Nevertheless, many patients fail to pursue fertility preservation options owing to two main barriers, time and cost. Of note, most procedures for fertility preservation are not covered by insurance in many countries.(6)

5. Conclusion

So it's fair to say that there have been substantial advances in fertility preservation in the last decade, but there still remain very significant gaps in our knowledge as to how best to proceed.

Patient selection remains a challenge, to be confident in offering treatment to those who need it and reassuring to those who do not. In this respect we have recently shown that serum AMH (anti müllerian hormone) predicts long-term ovarian function following chemotherapy in women with breast cancer. Indeed, in a multivariate analysis only AMH, but not age or FSH, remained a significant predictor.

This result, if confirmed, may allow a more individualised risk assessment based on the proposed treatment regime and a measure of the patient's ovarian reserve.

Improved cancer care associated with increased cure rates and long-term survival, coupled with advances in fertility treatment means that it is now imperative that fertility preservation is considered as part of the care offered to these patients. This can only be approached within a multidisciplinary setting. There are obvious challenges that still remain to be resolved, especially in the area of fertility preservation in prepubertal patients. These include ethical issues, such as valid consent and research in the area of tissue retrieval, cryopreservation and transplantation.

Long-term survival is expected in most women with cancer as a result of advances in cancer treatment. For young cancer survivors who have not completed their family, fertility is a crucial issue. Informed decision making regarding future fertility can lead to decreased patient regret and improved quality of life.

Use of less gonadotoxic regimens for adjuvant or neoadjuvant chemotherapy may be considered in young cancer patients with favourable tumors who are in their reproductive years. When there is a high risk of losing fertility with aggressive cancer treatment, currently available options for fertility preservation should be discussed. Embryo cryopreservation is a well-established technology and suitable for women who have a partner. Oocyte cryopreservation is an alternative option that can avoid ethical and legal issues (unlike embryo cryopreservation). However, neither embryo nor oocyte cryopreservation is a practical option for women who cannot delay cancer treatment. In addition, COS (Control Ovarian Stimulation) is required for both embryo and oocyte cryopreservation, and an increase in peak E2 levels with COS may accelerate tumour growth in some types of breast cancer with ERþ (estrogen-progestin receptors). The alternative COS strategy using tamoxifen or letrozole in conjunction with gonadotropin can suppress the elevation of E2 levels and may be considered for women with ERþ tumour in breast cancer.

Where embryo or oocyte cryopreservation is not indicated, cryopreservation of ovarian tissue can be a reasonable alternative, without the worry of delaying cancer treatment or increasing E2 levels. Fertility specialists should work closely with breast cancer treatment teams to provide options for fertility preservation before the initiation of cancer treatment in young women with breast cancer. A multidisciplinary program such as a breast cancer survivorship program will facilitate timely communications between oncologists and fertility specialists as well as effective transmission of information to health care providers and patients.(4)

In addition to developing techniques for preserving or restoring fertility, researchers should consider the long-term effects of such technologies, such as egg quality, healthy pregnancies and, most important, healthy babies.

The advisory panel also acknowledged the need to consider behavioural, cultural, religious, health disparities, ethical, legal and financial aspects of fertility preservation research.

6. References

[1] Green, DM; Whitton, JA; Stovall, M. et al. (2002). Pregnancy outcome of female survivors of childhood cancer: a report from the childhood Cancer Survivor Study. *Am J Obstet Gynecol*, vol. 187, Nº 4, pp. 1070-80.

[2] Jukkala, A.M.; Azuero, A.; McNees, P.; Bates, G.W.; Meneses, K.; (2010). Self-assessed knowledge of treatment and fertility preservation in young women with breast cancer. *Fertility and sterility,* vol. 94, nº 6, pp. 2396 – 2398, SN 0015-0282.

[3] Klock, S.C.; Zhang, J.X.; Kazer, R.R.; (2010). Fertility preservation for female cancer patients: early clinical experience. *Fertility and sterility.* Vol. 94, Nº 1, pp 149 – 155, SN 0015-0282.

[4] Kim, S.S.; Klemp, J.; Fabian, C.; (2011). Breast cancer and fertility preservation. *Fertility and sterility* . Vol. 95, Nº 5, pp 1535 – 1543, SN 0015-0282.

[5] Forman, E.J.; Anders, C.K.; Behera, M.A.; (2010). A nationwide survey of oncologists regarding treatment-related infertility and fertility preservation in female cancer patients. *Fertility and sterility.* Vol. 94, Nº5, pp 1652 – 1656, SN 0015-0282.

[6] Balthazar, U.; Fritz, M.A.; Mersereau, J.E.; (2011). Fertility preservation: a pilot study to assess previsit patient knowledge quantitatively. *Fertility and sterility* . Vol. 95, N° 6, pp 1913 - 1916, SN 0015-0282.

[7] Cruz, M.R.S.; Prestes, J.C.; Gimenes, D.L.; Fanelli, M. F.; (2010). Fertility preservation in women with breast cancer undergoing adjuvant chemotherapy: a systematic review. *Fertility and sterility.* Vol. 94, N° 1, pp 138 - 143 SN - 0015-0282.

[8] Lamar, C.A.; DeCherney, A.H.; (2009). Fertility preservation: state of the science and future research directions. *Fertility and sterility.* Vol. 91, N° 2, pp 316 - 319, SN 0015-0282.

[9] Oktay, K.; Sonmezer, M.; (2004). Ovarian tissue banking for cancer patients: Fertility preservation, not just ovarian cryopreservation. *Human Reproduction.* Vol 19, N° 3, pp 477-480.

[10] Ajala, T.; Rafi, J.; Larsen-Disney, P.; Howell R.; (2010). Fertility Preservation for Cancer Patients: A Review. *Obstetrics and Gynecology International.* Vol. 2010, article ID 160386.

[11] Kim S.; (2003). Ovarian tissue banking for cancer patients, To do or not to do?. *Human Reproduction.* Vol. 18, N° 9, pp 1759-1761.

[12] Meirow, D.; Hardan, I.; Dor J.; et al. (2008). Searching for evidence of disease and malignant cell contamination in ovarian tissue stored from hematologic cancer patients. *Human Reproduction.* Vol. 23, N° 5, pp. 1007-1013.

[13] Chambers, E.L.; Gosden, R.G.; Yap, C.; Picton, H.M.; (2010). In situ identification of follicles in ovarian cortex as a tool for quantifying follicle density, viability and developmental potential in strategies to preserve female fertility. *Human Reproduction.* Vol. 25, N° 10, pp. 2559-2568.

[14] Bedaiwy, M.A.; Falcone, T.; Goldberg, J.M.; Attaran, M.; Agarwal, A.; (2007). Fertility Preservation in Cancer Patients, In *Clinical Reproductive Medicine and Surgery,* Falcone, T. ; Hurd, W.W., pp 485-496, by Mosby, Inc. (Elsevier), ISBN 978-0-323-03309-1, Philadelphia (printed in China).

[15] Bedaiwy, M.A.; Falcone, T.; (2008). Fertility Preservation in Female and Male Cancer Patients, *Infertility and Assisted Reproduction,* Rizk, B.; Garcia-Velasco, J.; Sallam, H.; Makrigiannakis, A.; pp 706-716, by Cambridge University Press, ISBN 978-0-521-87379-6, United States of America.

[16] Forman E.J.; Anders, C.K.; Behera M.A.; (2010). A nation-vide survey of oncologist reagarding treatment-related infertility and fertility preservation in female cancer patients. *Fertility and Sterility.* Vol. 94, pp 1652-1656.

[17] *NHS National Institute for Clinical Excellence,* Clinical Guideline 11. 2004.

[18] Quinn, G.P.; Vadaparampil, S.T.; Gwede, C.K.; Miree, C.; King, L.M.; Clayton, H.B.; et al. (2007). Discussion of fertility preservation with newly diagnosed patients: Oncologists' views. *J Cancer Surviv.* Vol 1, pp 146-155.

[19] Cobo, A.; Domingo, J.; Pérez, S.; Crespo, J.; Remohí, J.; Pellicer, A.; (2008). Vitrification: an effective new approach to oocyte banking and preserving fertility in cancer patients. *Clin Transl Oncol.* Vol 10, N° 5, pp 268-73.

[20] British Fertility Society (2003). A strategy for fertility services for survivors of childhood cancer. *Human Fertility.* Vol.6,no.2, pp. A1–A40

[21] Sonoda, Y.; Abu-Rustum, N. R.; Gemignani, M. L.; et al. (2004) A fertility-sparing alternative to radical hysterectomy: how many patients may be eligible?. *Gynecologic Oncology*. Vol. 95, no. 3, pp. 534–538.

[22] Plante, M ; Renaud, M.-C. ; Hoskins, I. A. ; and Roy, M. (2005). Vaginal radical trachelectomy: a valuable fertility-preserving option in the management of early-stage cervical cancer. A series of 50 pregnancies and review of the literature. *Gynecologic Oncology*. vol. 98, no. 1, pp. 3–10.

[23] Brydoy, M.; Fossa, S. D. ; Klepp, O. ; et al. (2005) Paternity following treatment for testicular cancer. *Journal of the National Cancer Institute*. Vol. 97, no. 21, pp. 1580–1588.

[24] Huddart, R. A. ; Norman, A. ; Moynihan, C; .et al. (2005) Fertility, gonadal and sexual function in survivors of testicular cancer. *British Journal of Cancer*. Vol. 93, no. 2, pp. 200–207.

[25] Howell S.; and Shalet, S.; (1998). Gonadal damage from chemotherapy and radiotherapy. *Endocrinology and Metabolism Clinics of North America*. Vol. 27, no. 4, pp. 927–943.

[26] Schilsky, R. L. ; Lewis, B. J. ; Sherins, R. J.; and Young, R. C.; (1980) Gonadal dysfunction in patients receiving chemotherapy for cancer. *Annals of Internal Medicine*. Vol. 93, no. 1, pp. 109–114.

[27] Rivkees, S. A. and Crawford, J. D. (1988) The relationship of gonadal activity and chemotherapy-induced gonadal damage. *Journal of the American Medical Association*. Vol. 259, no. 14, pp. 2123–2125.

[28] Ferreyra, H. D.; (2009). Title of the conference *Fertility preservation in initial cervical cancer lesions*. La Rioja, Argentina. December 2009.

[29] Hahn, H.S.; Yoon, S.G.; Hong, J.S.; Hong, S.R.; Park, S.J.; Lim, J.Y.; Kwon, Y.S.; Lee, I.H.; Lim, K.T.; Lee, K.H.; Shim, J.U.; Mok, J.E.; Kim, T.J. (2009). Conservative treatment with progestin and pregnancy outcomes in endometrial cancer. *Int J Gynecol Cancer*. Vol 19, N° 6, pp 1068-73.

[30] Johnson, J.; Canning, J.; Kaneko, T.; Pru, J.K.; Tilly, J.L.; (2004) Germline stem cells and follicular renewal in the postnatal mammalian ovary. *Nature*. Vol 11, N° 428(6979), pp 145-50.

5

Dysmenorrhoea

Miguel Lugones Botell and Marieta Ramírez Bermúdez
University Polyclinic "26 de Julio",
Institute of Medical Sciences "Victoria de Giron", Havana,
Cuba

1. Introduction

It is about a colic pain located in the lower abdomen, it happens just before or during menstrual period and it usually comes with other symptoms: perspiration, tachycardia, sickness, vomits, diarrhea, etc and also It can cause lost of consciousness. This group of symptoms is usually called catamenial molimen.

2. Alternative names

Painful menstrual periods, menstrual colic. These terms are not very accepted scientifically and in general terms are more used for patients.

3. Frequency

It constitutes one of the main consultation reasons in young women population. Its frequency turns more significant when the gynecological and the axis hypophysis-hypothalamus-ovary maturation progresses. It is suffered by a 30 to 50% of the adolescents. Between the 10 and 15% of them are helpless of carrying out their school tasks.

4. Classification

The dysmenorrhoea is classified in primary and secondary. It is spoken of primary dysmenorrhoea in the cases of painful menstruations where there is not significant gynecologycal pathology. It appears for the first time from 6 to 12 months after having happened the menarche when the ovulatory cycles are already well established because this is a dysfunction of women that ovulate.

The secondary dysmenorrhoea is product of an existent pelvic affection and it is characterized because it begins several years after the menarche and the pain last more during the menstruation. The most frequent causes of secondary dysmenorrhoea are: endometriosis (33,5%), pelvic inflammatory illness, uterine myoma, uterine polyps, cervical stenosis, pelvic adherences, use of intra-uterine devices, congenital anomalies of the development of the genital tract (fundamentally the obstructive ones), and ovary cysts.

Membranous dysmenorrhoea as some authors denominate it -, consists on the presence of intense colic caused by the step of endometrial tissue (uterine cover) through the not distended uterine neck and it is not very common.

5. Etiology

Dysmenorrhoea cause was ignored during a lot of time. Pickles was the first one in suggesting that it was caused by a "menstrual stimulant" and later he discovered that it was a prostaglandin mixture (PG) E2 and F2.

There are a lot of works that link the dysmenorrhoea to the action of the prostaglandins; their levels are increased in cases of dysmenorrhoea, myomas, etc. The prostaglandins F2 and the prostaglandins E2 are so much in high concentrations in the secretor endometrium and in the menstrual fluid of women with primary dysmenorrhoea. The prostaglandins F2 is a potent oxytocic uteroconstrictor; when it is administrated inside the uterus it produces an intense pain like the one that happens in the dysmenorrhoea and occasionally, menstrual bleeding. The role of the prostaglandins E2 is less clear, but it could increase the sensibility of the nervous terminations.

The reason of the increase of the values of the prostaglandins in the primary dysmenorrhoea is not very well-known. The primary dysmenorrhoea happens almost exclusively in ovulatory cycles and it is known that the steroid hormones of the ovary affect the uterine contractility. However, the existence of any abnormality has not been demonstrated in the hormonal values of women with primary dysmenorrhoea, neither the exact relationship between progesterone and primary dysmenorrhoea.

It has also been proved that the exogenous supply of prostaglandins causes contractions of the myometrium and the increase of the dose entails associated symptoms: vomits, uneasiness, diarrhea.

Other factors related to the etiology of the primary dysmenorrhoea are the uterine synthesis of leukotriene, the increased secretion of vasopressin, the endothelin or the activator factor of the platelets.

Psychological and cervical factors were considered before as important etiopathogenic factors, they have lost a lot of value as fundamental cause of the dysmenorrhoea, being valued at the moment as preponderant factors, according to what we already pointed out; the role of the hormones and of the prostaglandins.

Nevertheless, we should not stop recognizing there are patients that somatize more than others. It has also been studied groups of adolescents and we can also observe that those with more crises in their life experimented more marked symptoms.

The emotional reaction in front of the menstrual period has aspects of cultural nature that determine different attitudes we can not obviate.

6. Clinical manifestations

In the primary dysmenorrhoea the pain settles -as we already pointed out-, just before or during the first moments the menstruation appears. Its time of duration varies from 2-3 hours up to 1 day and with less frequency, between 2 and 3 days. There are cases in which the pain can begin between 2 and 3 days before the menstruation, but it is uncommon, it is usually of colic type, in hypogastrium, it is irradiated to lumbar region and both thighs. Gradations of intensity exist as well as associated syndromes.

There are some differences in the clinical manifestations between the primary and secondary dysmenorrhoea, for example, in secondary dysmenorrhoea, the beginning of the sintomatology is after the first two years of having happened the menarche and the symptoms can appear days before the menstruation and after having happened this one, its duration is usually longer, contrary to the primary one in which we already pointed out, its beginning is in the first two years of having happened the menarche, the symptoms are presented almost with the menstruation and its duration is briefer.

Besides the presence of some discoveries like inflammatory processes, endometriosis, etc., will differentiate the secondary dysmenorrhoea of the primary one.

CHARACTERISTICS	**PRIMARY**	**SECONDARY**
Moment of the cycle	Lightly before or during the menstruation. There is more pain during the menstruation.	It doesn't usually limit to the menstruation. The pain is not always more intense with the menstruation.
Relationship with menstrual bleeding.	The pain is related with the first day of having bled.	The pain is not related with the first day of having bled.
Characteristic of the pain.	it is the same in all menstruations.	It tends to get worst with the time.
Duration of the pain.	24 to 72 hours	4 to 6 days
Age of beginning.	Adolescence (Generally 1 to 2 years after the menarche)	Women older than 20 years (among 20 -30 years in endometriosis), among 30-40 years in adenomyosis.
Associated symptoms	Sikness, vomits, diarrhea, migraine, depression.	Infertility, metrorrhagia, dyspareunia
Gynecological antecedents	There are not antecedents.	Some antecedent exists.
Gynecological exam.	Negative.	Discovery of: Palpable Tumoration Fixed uterine retroversion. Old painful. Painful Uterosacros. Presence of uterine dispositive

Table 1. Comparison between the primary and secondary dysmenorrhoea

7. Differential diagnosis

It is very important to differentiate the primary dysmenorrhoea of the secondary one. A good questioning should be carried out; it allows us to discard the presence or not of causes related to the physiological menstrual cycle or causes unaware to this cycle. Later a meticulous and correct gynecological physical exam will supplement the elements to make the differentiation.

Among the most frequent causes of secondary dysmenorrhoea -as we pointed out-, is the one caused by endometriosis, that represents 33,5% of the causes of secondary dysmenorrhoea. It is suspected when:

a. We find painful nodules in the uterosacral ligaments in the pelvic exam.
b. When the pain becomes progressive in each menstruation.
c. When there is poor answer to the treatment.

Other important causes are the intra-uterine devices, which are sometimes ignored by patients, those that unchain reactions mediated by the prostaglandins and the uterine myomas.

8. Treatment: General considerations

The dysmenorrhoea has been treated from the symptomatic, endocrine and surgical point of view; we will analyze these treatments.

It is very important to offer to the patient an explanation of her affection and its possible causes after being defined if the affection is type primary or secondary one. In not few cases, mainly in those that the dysmenorrhoea process is manifested with light pain, just the information of the natural phenomena of the menstruation -psychotherapy - is enough to make the patients feel better.

As we already pointed out, it is very important to carry out a good questioning not only to establish the diagnosis and to specify if it is a primary or secondary dysmenorrhoea, but also to know some characteristics of the patient's personality, if she has received previous treatments and in this case, to be able to specify which ones have been indicated and by whom.

The treatment of the dysmenorrhoea crisis depends on its seriousness. Once initiated the pain it is necessary to assist to its natural evolution. Generally intense dysmenorrhoea responds to the local application of heat and light analgesic, sedative or antispasmodics. Physical exercise is usually a benefit.

The rehabilitative treatment of the dysmenorrhoea has been recommended Independently of the classical treatment based on anti-inflammatory non steroid, inhibitors of prostaglandins, norms of intestinal hygiene, to prevent the constipation and local heat, It will be summarized at the end of this work.

A practical focus for the initial handling of the treatment is presented in figure I.

As we can see in figure 1, the main strategy to establish the treatment consists on defining pretty well if it is a primary or secondary dysmenorrhoea.

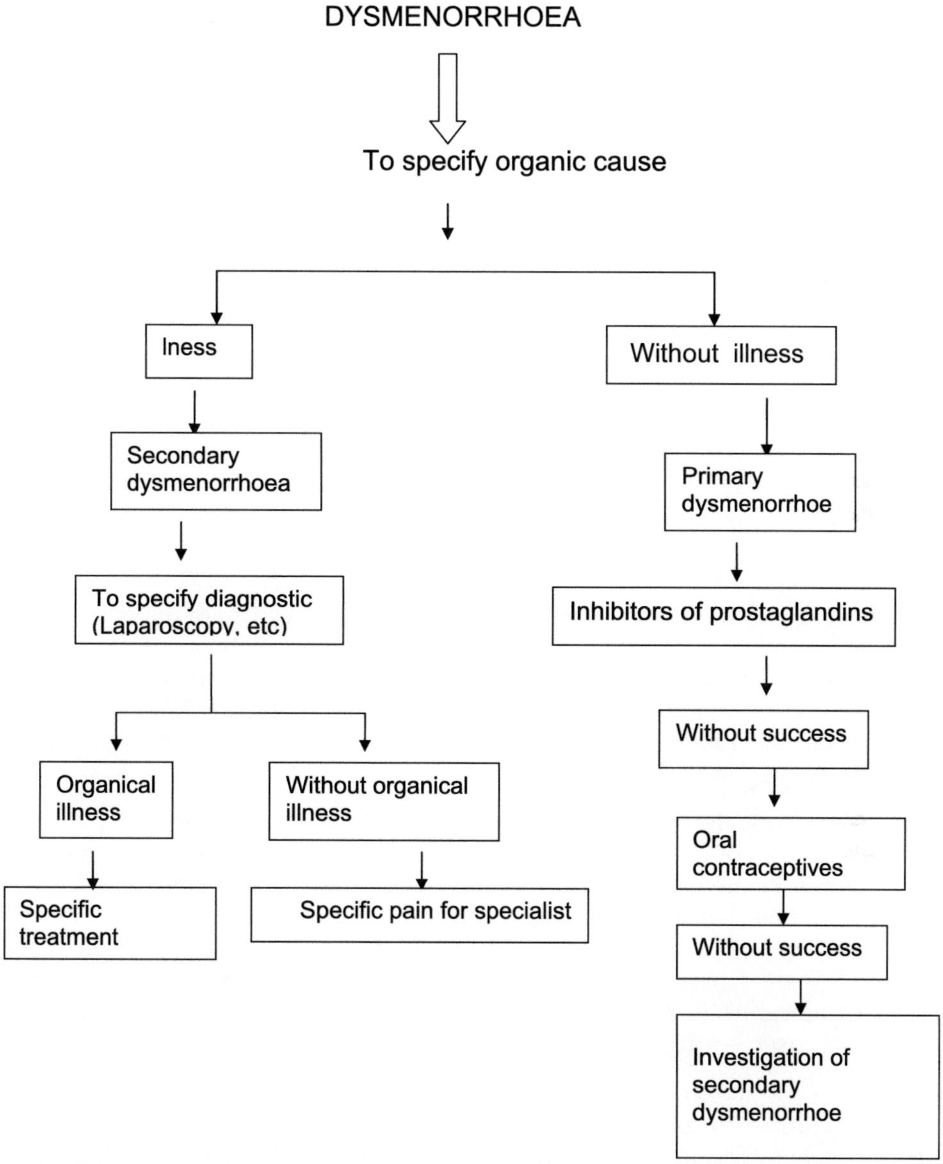

Fig. 1. Approach for the treatment of the dysmenorrhoea.

9. Considerations of treatment

a. Symptomatic treatment

We already pointed out that the observation of the intensity of the pain, its limitations and the presence or not of associated syndromes will give us the guidelines to establish, when classifying the dysmenorrhoea according to its grade. It is always convenient to keep in mind a group of general measures- already distinguished- like sedative ones, antispasmodics, physical exercises, etc.

b. Hormonal treatment

Oral contraceptives are very effective and they constitute the chosen treatment in women that require contraception and they don't have contraindications. The explanation of the observed benefits with oral contraceptives is the decrease of the prostaglandins synthesis associated to an atrophic endometrium; it diminishes the menstrual flow and therefore the prostaglandins. Oral contraceptives are a good choice: It is combined the contraception with a beneficial effect on the dysmenorrhoea, menstrual flow and menstrual irregularities.

When inhibiting the ovulation, the prostaglandin content in the menstrual liquid diminishes below the normal figures and decreases its contractile effect on the uterine musculature.

The effectiveness of the synthetic progestogens is smaller than oral contraceptives. The possibility to carry out a hormonal treatment with progesterone derives (medroxyprogesterone or dydrogesterone 5-10 mg/days) can be considered during the last 10-12 days of the cycle. At the present time most of the progestational drugs are used in form of oral contraceptives and we should remember that the use of the pill during 21 days to control one or two days of dysmenorrhoea is not recommended if contraception is not required.

c. Inhibitors of prostaglandins

The coming of the inhibitors of synthetase of PG constitutes a new dimension and with success in its treatment. It has been studied 5 main groups of inhibitors of the synthetase of prostaglandins and clinical studies show that these drugs relieve the symptomatology of dismenorrhoea. The compounds that inhibit the biosynthesis of the PG can act in 2 different places in the cascade of the arachidonic acid through the inhibition of the enzymatic system. The inhibitors are divided into 2 different types:

Type I. Acts inhibiting the recurrent synthesis from the endoperoxide to the cyclooxygenase level. Some examples of inhibitors of type I are the indomethacin and the mefenamic acid. Among the anti-inflammatory non steroids families we can find the group of acetic acid, one example of this one is the indomethacin, this group is associated to a lot of collateral effects and they are not drugs for choice for dysmenorrhoea treatment. The drugs (mefenamic acid, flufenamic acid) are extremely effective. Fenemates act as inhibitors of the synthetase and they have an antagonistic action on the receivers of the prostaglandins. Also Ibuprofen, ketoprofen, naproxen belong to this group, are very effective.

Type II. They act on the enzymes that disintegrate the recurrent endoperoxides. Type II are the p-cloromercuribenzoate and the butyrophenone phenylbutazone, these don't inhibit the cyclooxygenase and they allow the production of recurrent endoperoxides, which are potent uterotonic.

In general terms, the different inhibitors of the synthetase prostaglandins are similar and there are not studies that compare them in an effective way. All these drugs are useful and they cause relief of the dysmenorrhoea symptoms in most of sick people.

The collateral effects of the inhibitors and antagonistic of the prostaglandins are relatively light and quite passable. Migraine, digestive symptoms, blurred vision, vertigo and erythema are pointed out. Women with antecedents of gastrointestinal ulcer should not take these drugs. Sometimes, the patients describe a disorientation sensation and others of sleepiness, sickness and edginess. We can not forget the nephrotoxicity potential of these drugs.

Initially, it was thought that the best effects in the inhibitors of the prostaglandins were achieved with the administration 2-3 days before the menstruation, to reduce the prostaglandin levels in tissues before the endometrial collapse. Fortunately the studies have proved that the effectiveness of the treatment is the same when the bled begins, therefore, the possibility of ingestion of these agent decreases in the first stage of the pregnancy. Another benefit of the inhibition of prostaglandins is the decrease of the lost of blood during the menstruation.

d. Presacral neurectomy

The presacral neurectomy or sympathectomy constitutes a rational and effective procedure in patients that suffer intense dysmenorrhoea and don't respond to the treatment. Since, although it alleviates totally or almost the pain is a bigger surgical intervention--with non despicable risks--, and there is not guarantee of a beneficent answer, it is a method in disuse. The resection of the uterosacral ligaments and the lumbar and ovarian sympathectomy are abandoned technics.

e. Hysterectomy

In some patients with secondary dysmenorrhoea- due to very extensive endometriosis and rebellious to treatments, tumorous like uterine myomas, etc- will be suitable the total abdominal hysterectomy.

Grade	Clinical Manifestation	Treatment
I	Light dysmenorrhoea. Without systemic symptoms. Without interference in the activities	Education Menstrual calendar. Analgesic. Oral contraceptives
II	Moderate dysmenorrhoea. Without systemic or scarce symptoms. It interferes the activities, partially.	Education. Menstrual calendar Ibuprofen 400 mg every 8 hours or sour mefenamic 500 beginning mg and then 250 mg every 6 hours.
III	Intense dysmenorrhoea. There are systemic symptoms. It interferes the activities	Sodium naproxen in suppositories 500 beginning mg and then 250 mg every 6 hours.

Table 2. Behavior according to the grade of intensity of the dysmenorrhoea

Light dysmenorrhoea

The treatment is based on the patient's education, the use of menstrual calendar, analgesic and oral contraceptives.

Moderate dysmenorrhoea

Education is also important. It is allowed to increase the aspirin dose to 500 mg every 6 hours. Antispasmodic and muscle relaxants are useful. Progestogens has demonstrated their effectiveness in the second half of the cycle. It is insisted a lot in the effectiveness of the ibuprofen in this stage.

Severe dysmenorrhoea

Maintain the general educational measures, the use of the calendar, etc, we pointed out in the previous square.

Many authors insist in the advantage of the sodium naproxen in suppositories 500 mg. at the beginning and then 250 mg every 6 hours.

Secondary dysmenorrhoea

In general terms, this type of dysmenorrhoea gets better with the specific treatment of the underlying cause.

9.1 Rehabilitation

It is another alternative form of treatment that some authors recommend independently that it is carried out previously the signal therapy.

9.2 Kinesitherapy

Its objective is to get relaxation of the back musculature, and to strengthen the different muscular groups with the purpose of avoiding antalgic postures that could cause, secondarily, contractions in adductors muscles and in the lumbar region. It is proposed the following guide of exercises following Beare and Myers:

1. Balance of the back. It seeks to stretch the paravertebral muscles, of the back and neck, as well as those of the buttocks. To get this, the patient in supine position and relaxed, will take the knees to the chest placing her hands intertwined in the hollow popliteal. In that position, she will practice from five to 10 slow swinging movements toward before and behind, from the buttocks until the neck.
2. Sit down partially. Its purpose is to strengthen the abdominal muscles. The patient in supine position with bent knees and leaning feet on the floor will contract the abdominal musculature and bend slowly the trunk until being held to their knees with extended arms. She will stay in that position for five seconds, returning then, slowly, to the departure position. She will repeat the exercise from five to 10 times.
3. Basculation of the pelvis. Its objective is to strengthen the abdominal and lumbar musculature. The departure position is the one of supine with bent knees and feet on the floor with crisscross hands behind the nape. Then, she will contract, firmly the muscles of the buttocks and abdomen, pressing the low part of the back against the support plane. She will maintain the contraction during five seconds and she will relax later. She will repeat the exercise from five to 10 times.
4. Kegel's exercises. They are good to strengthen the muscles of the floor of the pelvis. The patient can start from sitting or upright position. She is asked to contract the musculature of the floor of the pelvis strongly (like to interrupt the urinal flow) during five seconds, relaxing next and repeating the exercise 10 times. This exercise will be carried out several times a day. Then, the patient in supine position with a pillow under the hollow popliteal and crossed legs, will be requested to press the buttocks and contract the anus (like to avoid the defecation). The knees should remain firmly pressed during 5 seconds; then the patient should relax them and repeat that at least 10 times.

9.3 Microwaves

It is well-known that electromagnetic waves of high frequency produce heat in deep tissues, especially in those that have high content of water. The muscle, the interstitial liquid and the blood warm in a more selective way. This has a favorable effect on the dysmenorrhoea when improving the flow of blood through the myometrium, being eliminated in this way, the prostaglandins producers of the pain. Nevertheless, and to assure a bigger penetration, you could opt for a therapy with pulsatile microwaves with irradiator of round field R, inserting cushions of sand so that the field, homogeneously concentrated, can act with more intensity and more deeply.

An intermediate level of power of 45 watts will be used. The application will be made at abdominal level and with the patient in supine or lateral position. The number of sessions will be in function of the intensity of the pain. It will be enough, in general, with one or two days for menstrual cycle, being carried out the application in the moment of appearance of the symptoms. The treatment will be continued during 6-7 cycles, been proved that in the following menstrual cycles after the application of the treatment the obtained improvement is the same. As the existence of metallic objects in the place of the treatment is a formal contraindication for the application of microwaves, it will be contraindicated in carriers of intra-uterine devices or others metallic implants.

9.4 TENS

The electric transcutaneous nervous stimulation has been described as an effective and innocuous method for the relief of pain in primary dysmenorrhoea. It is used Impulses between 0, 2 and 1 ms and a frequency of 70-100 Hz (11). The intensity will be adapted to the patient's sensibility, trying to arrive to 40-50 MA. The application will be carried out on inferior abdominal region, sacroiliac region and the last two lumbar levels.

9.5 Relaxation techniques

The most used technique is the progressive relaxation of Jacobson, it considers that emotional experiences can represent a predisposing factor in the appearance of dysmenorrhoea, due to the existent nexus between personal experience and muscular tensions (uterine, abdominal, lumbar and adductors, in this case). The relaxation session will last one hour, it starts taking a progressive and continuous conscience of the different areas of the body, until the patient gets to the so called differential relaxation, looking for the minimum of necessary tension to carry out an act.

10. Comments

It won't always be necessary to make use of all the therapeutic methods described previously. Everything will depend on the severity of the manifestation and on the acceptance of the patient to some of the signalled methods.

11. References

[1] Abraham GE. Primary dysmenorrhea. Clin Obstet Gynecol 1978;21:139-45.

[2] Andersch B, Milsom I. An epidemiologic study of young women with dysmenorrhea. Am J Obstet Gynecol 1982;3:71-94.

[3] Arbués Lacadena J. Dismenorrea. Protocolos de Obstetricia y Ginecología. Madrid, SEGO 2001; Proto A2/prot 2-56 htm.

[4] Cavanaugh R: Nongynecologic causes of unexplained lower abdominal pain in adolescents girl. Clínical pediatrics.1996; 35 (7): 25-35.

[5] Duarte Contreras A: Ginecología de la niña y de la adolescente. Ed. Salvat. España. 1988: 93-101.

[6] Kennedy ST. Primary dysmenorrhea. Lancet 1997;349: 1116-7.

[7] Lawlor CH: Primary dismenorrhea. J of adoles. Heath care. 1981; 208: 97.

[8] Lérida Ortega M. A. Platero Rico D. Ponce Castro J. Ávila Ávila C. J. Tratamiento rehabilitador de la dismenorrea primaria. REHABILITACIÓN. 1999; 33(5): 335-38

[9] Levy S Bárbara MD: Causas diversas de dolor pélvico. En: Steege J. MD: Dolor pélvico crónico. México. Interamericana. 1999. 150- 153.

[10] Machado HM, Rodríguez PO: Dolor pelviano en la adolescente. En: Jorge Peláez Mendoza. Ginecología Infanto Juvenil. Salud Reproductiva del adolescente. Científico Técnica. La Habana. 1999. 122-127.

[11] Marc R Laufer, Donald P. Goldstein: Dismenorrea, dolor pélvico y syndrome premenstrual. En: Jean Herriot Emans MD: Ginecología en Pediatría y la adolescencia. México. Interamericana. 2000. 282-286.

[12] Pickles VR: A plain muscle stimulant in the menstruan. Nature 1957; 180: 1198

[13] Speroff L, Glass RH, Kase NG. Trastornos menstruales. En: Speroff L, Glass RH, Kase NG. Editores. Endocrinología ginecológica e infertilidad. Buenos Aires, Madrid, Waverly Hispánica Organón 2000;557-73.

[14] Rees M. Dysmenorrhea. Br J Obstet Gynaecol 1998;95:833-5.

[15] Sundell G, Milsom I, Andersch B. Factors influencing the prevalence and severity of dysmenorrhea in young women. Br J Obstet Gynaecol 1990;97:588-94.

[16] Zeiguer BK: Trastornos del ciclo menstrual. Dismenorrea. En su: Ginecología Infanto Juvenil. Argentina. Panamericana. 1993. Segunda edición. 303-305.

6

Abortions in Low Resource Countries

Robert J.I. Leke and Philip Njotang Nana
University of Yaounde I,
Cameroon

1. Introduction

Abortion is the termination of pregnancy within the first half of pregnancy (WHO) or before 28 completed weeks within the context of developing countries. However, fetuses weighing less than 500 gms 0r less than 900gms in the developed or developing counties constitute abortion. [1, 2, 3]

The tabulated estimates of the frequency of abortions by WHO (1994) showed that there were about 20 million illegal abortions performed each year and the greatest majority of these unsafe abortions occur in developing countries and particularly countries in which abortion law was restricted and illegal. Incidentally these were also the countries that presented a lack of supplies and commodities as well as insufficient trained personnel. In these countries many maternal deaths due to complications of abortions are either not registered or deliberately concealed. [2, 3, 4]

2. Clinical classifications

Clinical classification divides abortions into different categories that determine their prognosis and different therapeutic approaches. Abortions are spontaneous or induced, the spontaneous type accounting for 10-15% of all known or suspected pregnancies. The true incidence especially in developing countries may not be known because of the difficulty to recognize early pregnancies and their losses. The commonest cause of spontaneous abortion is chromosomal anomalies and the most common of these anomalies is Autosomal trisomy occurring in about 51.9% of the anomalies. The second most common type of chromosomal anomaly in spontaneously aborted fetuses is monosomy x (45, xo) and occurs in 18.9% of aborted fetuses. (Scott 1986). The rates of spontaneous abortions are relatively constant between populations and are rarely the cause of severe abortion complications and maternal death.

The clinical categories of spontaneous abortions are the following:

- Threatened abortion
- Inevitable or Eminent Abortion
- Incomplete abortion
- Complete Abortion
- Missed Abortion
- Habitual Abortion

- **Induced abortions:** This is abortion carried out in an environment inappropriate for service delivery and/ or by persons and providers in-experienced in abortion care delivery and without adequate infection prevention measures. Induced abortion can also be carried out by trained abortion providers within appropriate service. Induced abortion can be sub-classed into:
- **Therapeutic abortion:** This is abortion conducted for medical indications either to save the life of the woman and preserve the physical and mental health, foetal malformation incompatible with extra uterine life (anencephaly, multi-organ malformations, transposition of the great blood vessels, active rubella infection in early pregnancy etc) and rape as spelled out in the penal code in its articles 337-340 for Cameroon. These indications though restricted in our environment and the developing countries are still underutilized. Other legal indications for abortion include economic or social factors or pregnancy resulting from incest. The Cameroonian law permits marriage of first cousins. Therapeutic abortion is also indicated in situations of missed abortion or blighted ovum.
- **Clandestine or unsafe voluntary abortion:** This is abortion carried out by unqualified, non competent staff, in an inappropriate environment and without infection prevention. Complications of such procedures occur latter and the patients are usually admitted 2-3 days after the procedure.
- **Septic abortions:** This is usually a consequence of unsafe abortion. In the study on the Assessment of the National Magnitude of abortion and direct cost evaluation in Cameroon 23.1% of all abortions were induced [3, 11]. This figure is just the tip of the iceberg as most risk free induced abortions carried out by qualified health care providers are complication free. A number of septic abortions may be a consequence of a spontaneous abortion.

Abortion remains a major public health problem in Sub-Saharan Africa. When an unmarried young woman becomes pregnant in a low resource environment she faces a difficult dilemma: if she decides to carry the pregnancy to term, this is usually characterized by poor antenatal care and obstructive complications. Some 40% of all abortions are high risk and unsafe with one woman in 400 dying from complications. Hospital studies in Sub-Saharan Africa show that 30-40% of maternal deaths are due to complications of unsafe abortion. It is now accepted that about ninety percent of abortion complications occur in developing countries with risk of death in Africa being one in 150 cases [3]. It is also accepted that about 50% of all pregnancies are not planned and 25% of these pregnancies are unwanted and this explains the high number of about 100.000 women who die from complications of abortions in developing countries every year. In Africa south of the Sahara, other major factors contribute to the high numbers of death due to abortions and these include: low prevalence rate of modern contraception (13% in Cameroon) with a high unmet need for family planning(44% in Cameroon)(DHS 2010). This is also coupled with low education of adolescent girls and women as well as early and forced teenage marriages.

Besides there is cruel need for services for risk groups like adolescents, and unmarried mothers and to these we must add the role played by restrictive abortion laws that still exist and prevail in the region. The restrictive laws on abortion do not permit adolescents and women to terminate an unwanted pregnancy under safe and legal conditions. Most countries of Francophone Africa still respect and use the 1920 anti Abortion French law and consequently most termination of pregnancy in the region is done by untrained personnel and in very unsafe conditions. [6, 7, 8]

3. Reproductive rights of women, adolescents and abortion laws

Though most developing countries still have restrictive laws towards safe abortion services, they are signatories to a number of international treaties and laws as concerns the reproductive rights of the woman and the adolescent. Reproductive health can be defined as a state of complete physical, mental and social well-being and not merely the absence of disease or infirmity, in all matters relating to the reproductive system and to its functions and processes. Reproductive health therefore implies that people are able to have a satisfying and safe sex life, which they have the capability to reproduce, and the freedom to decide when and how often to do so. Men and women therefore have a right to be informed and have access to safe, effective, affordable and acceptable methods of family planning of their choice, as well as other methods of their choice for fertility regulation which are not against the law. It also implies that couples have the right of access to appropriate health care services that will enable women go through pregnancy safely and provide the best chances of having a healthy infant. [9]

The International Planned Parenthood Federation (IPPF) has produced a formal statement declaring women and men´s sexual and reproductive rights to be essential components of human rights. The IPPF rights are developed based on the international human rights agreements and consist of 12 principles.

The laws on abortion are described in a number of documents such as:

- International treaties, conventions, agreements and covenants: In principle, international treaties, when ratified by a country, supersede the national law. This is not the case in most of our developing countries.
- National laws (The national medical ethics code): The lack of clarity in many laws is a serious dysfunction and Health care providers´ apprehensions cause them to decline involvement, so that women resort to illegal and unsafe practices in cases where the law actually allows procedures by skilled and qualified providers.
- Customary laws, Islamic (Shar´ah) laws.

40.5% of the world´s population lives in countries with restrictive law on abortion, though they are signatories to most of the treaties and conventions on the rights of the woman. However, abortion is legalized for the following indications in the world, socioeconomic factors (14 nations, 20.7%), mental health (20 nations, 2.7% of world´s population), physical health (35 nations, 10.1%), and safe life or prohibited (72 nations, 26%) [10].

4. Abortion complications [5, 8, 12, 13, 14]

Studies carried out within the countries have shown abortion to be associated with a number of complications. Complications of abortions are a leading cause of morbidity and mortality of women in low resource countries.

The tables below highlight some of these complications.

Complications	Frequency	Percent
Hemorrhage	30	34
Cervical Laceration	20	22.7
Vaginal Vault Tear	9	10.2
Cervical Burns	6	6.8
Septicaemia	6	6.8
Uterine Perforation	4	4.6
Pelvic Abscess	4	4.6
Pyometria	3	3.4
Intestinal Perforation	2	2.3
Rectal Perforation	2	2.3
Bladder Perforation	2	2.4
Total	**88**	**100**

Source: Leke, Tikum (1991).

Table 1. Common complications associated with suspected or induced abortions.

Medical complications of abortion	Spontaneous abortion	Safe induced abortion	Unsafe induced abortion
Haemorrhage	mild	mild	Moderate -severe
Infection	mild	mild	Severe
Internal trauma	mild	mild	Severe
Hospitalization	short	short	Prolonged
Morbidity, Infertility	low	low	Moderate –severe
Maternal mortality	low	low	High

Table 2. Abortion consequences, Spontaneous, Safe induced and Unsafe induced abortions.

The table clearly demonstrates that induced abortion is usually associated with severe morbidity such as haemorrhage, anaemia, infection, fistulae, infertility, ectopic pregnancy and upper and lower genital tract lacerations. These complications are still commonly seen in our environment today since the law remains restrictive and adolescents as well as single mothers are most affected by the need for abortion services.

In sub-saharan Africa reports from hospital studies suggest that induced abortion is probably increasing (Mbango) [13].Besides many of the patients with abortions are young, nulliparous and single but women of all reproductive ages, both married and single, suffer from the consequences of unsafe abortions.

In Yaoundé, Cameroon Leke and Tikum [6] reported that induced abortion was fifty times more likely to cause maternal death than a normal delivery in the same environment. They also reported that complications of induced abortion contributed to 34.6% of maternal mortality in their hospital.

A similar experience has been reported in Addis Ababa where a community based study showed that 24% of all maternal deaths directly related to pregnancy were attributed to complications of induced abortions.

QUANTITY OF PUS	FREQUENCY	%
<5000ml	14	36
500 - 999ml	7	18
1000 - 1999ml	14	36
2000 - 6000ml	4	10
TOTAL	**39**	**100**

Nana P.N. et Al (2005)

Table 3. Quantity of pus collection.

Peritonitis is a common complication of induced abortion in low resource countries. The above table reports on the amount of pus collection seen at laparotomy in women operated for post abortum peritonitis.The volume of pus found at surgery ranged from 20-6000ml with a mean of 1206ml. Abscess collection was seen in the pouch of Douglas, paracolic gutters and the sub-splenic angle.

ORGAN	FREQUENCY	%
The Uterus	27	54
Small intestine	5	19
Sigmoid colon	2	8
Bladder	1	4
Omemtum	10	38
No lesion found	23	46

Nana P.N. et Al (2005)

Table 4. Traumatic lesions found at surgery

Complications of induced abortion normally include damage to other organs. In 54% of the patients there was perforation on the uterus. The uterus was not perforated in 46% of the cases. Abdominal viscera were damaged in 18 of the 27 patients with uterine perforation. In two patients the small intestine and / or omentum herniated into the uterine rent. The length of the rent varied between 1 and 10 cm, involving the fundus, posterior, anterior and lateral walls of the uterus. In six of the fifty patients the fundus and / or the corpus was gangrenous. There were more than one perforation of the small intestine in two of the five affected cases. One of the two patients with a rent on the sigmoid colon required the presence of a visceral surgeon. The patient had a segmentary resection of the colon and colostomy with eventual end to end anastomosis.

Tables 5 and 6 clearly shows that unplanned pregnancies account for 38.7% of all patients presenting with incomplete abortion. A similar percentage carries had an in the complete (38.1%) carried induced abortion after 12 weeks of pregnancy. Unmet contraceptive needs coupled with lack of knowledge or family planning, financial constraints and lack of a male support all favour women to seek induced abortion.

Nature	Frequency	Percent
Wanted	245	61.3
Unwanted	155	38.7
Total	**400**	**100**

Report Leke et al (2009)

Table 5. Nature of pregnancy (Wanted/Unwanted)

Gestation (Weeks)	frequency	percent
3-12	229	61.9
13-20	109	29.5
21+	32	8.6
Total	**370**	**100**

Report Leke et al (2009)

Table 6. Distribution of patients by gestational Age.

5. Methods of pregnancy termination in low resource countries

The method used in terminating a pregnancy in low resource countries is provider dependent and consist of the following:

Individual: This is done through the ingestion of different concoctions such as whisky, blue detergent, medications contraindicated in pregnancy and the use of potassium permanganate. In a study carried out in the Tiko and Limbe towns Leke et al, reported that the following substances were used for pregnancy termination, native medication 33%, pharmaceutical products 29%, D&C 21%. The woman was the provider in 40 % and the General Practitioner in 15% of cases.

Traditional doctors/ non qualified providers: Several types of concoctions are administered either orally or as vaginal pessaries. Sometimes different instruments such as hysterometers, sponge forceps, cassava stems etc are used to initiate the procedure as seen in Figure 1 below.

Among the several substances used by traditional doctors and non qualified providers to induce abortions are the below. Some of these substances certainly contain prostaglandin-like or oxytocin-like substances that initiate contractions. A greater number are using Misoprostol since its introduction into the list of essential drugs.

The below picture on figure 2 shows a woman operated for suspected abdominal pregnancy at term. Per operatively, the foetus was found to float in the abdomen, the placenta was adherent to the omentum, and other scarred wounds from perforation were seen on the uterus. It is possible the Placenta villi migrated through the perforation to become adherent on the omentum. Secondarily, the uterus ruptured and the foetus continued to grow within the abdominal cavity. After surgery, patient acknowledged she terminated a 2nd trimester abortion that was complicated and had uterine evacuation twice. The rent was repaired, tubes ligated and placenta delivered by partial omentectomy.

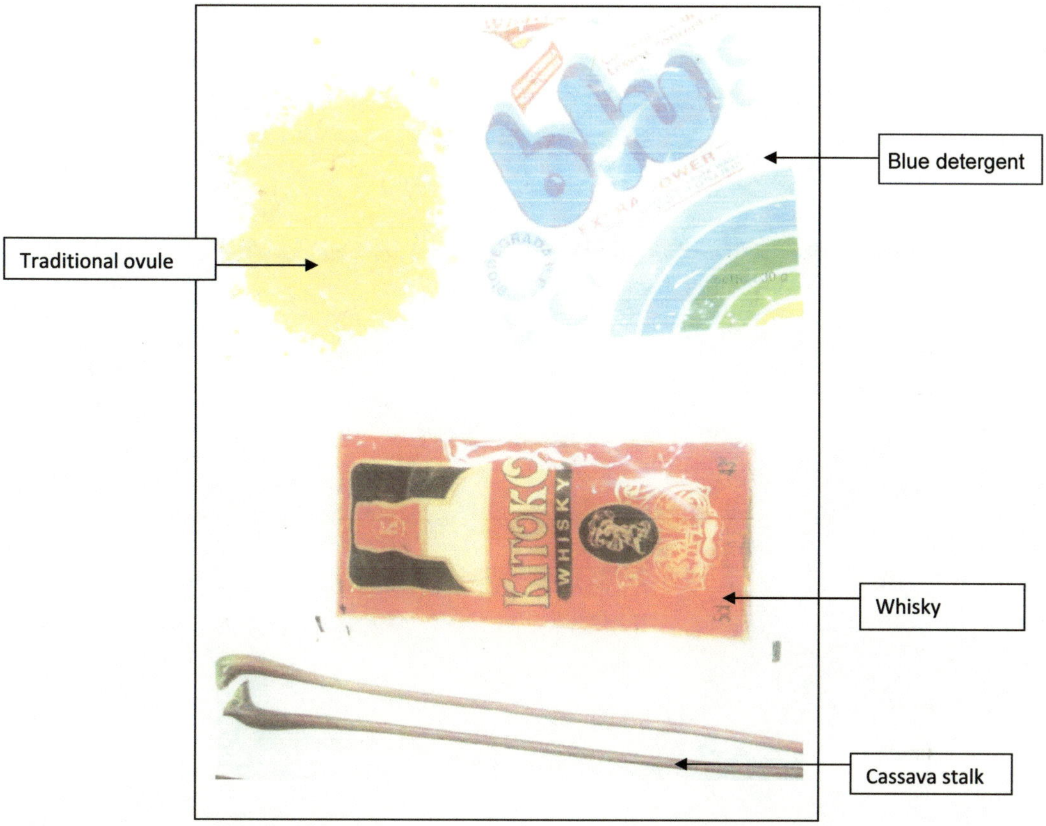

Fig. 1. Concoctions and instruments.

Nurses and Midwives: Here attempts are made to carry out procedures seen within the hospital in unsafe environment and sometimes not taking into consideration the gestational age of the pregnancy. Methods like amniotomy, dilatation and curettage, medical abortion with misoprostol and oxcytocin are utilised.

Doctors: Even though most African countries still use the old techniques of dilatation and curettage to evacuate the uterus for incomplete abortions or pregnancy termination, a gradual and progressive increase in the number of Doctors and midwives trained in the use of the manual vacuum aspirator is increasing in the milieu. This is the advised method for pregnancy termination as most epidemiological studies have shown that vacuum aspiration (electric or mechanical) is the safest, simplest, economic and effective means of inducing first trimester abortion as well as treating first trimester incomplete abortion.

Advantages of the manual vacuum aspirator.

- Reduction of post evacuation complications,
- Increased access to service.

- Shortened duration of hospitalization.
- Reduction in abortion service cost
- Reduced utilization of scarce resources.
- Technique easy to learn and use by several categories of health personnel.

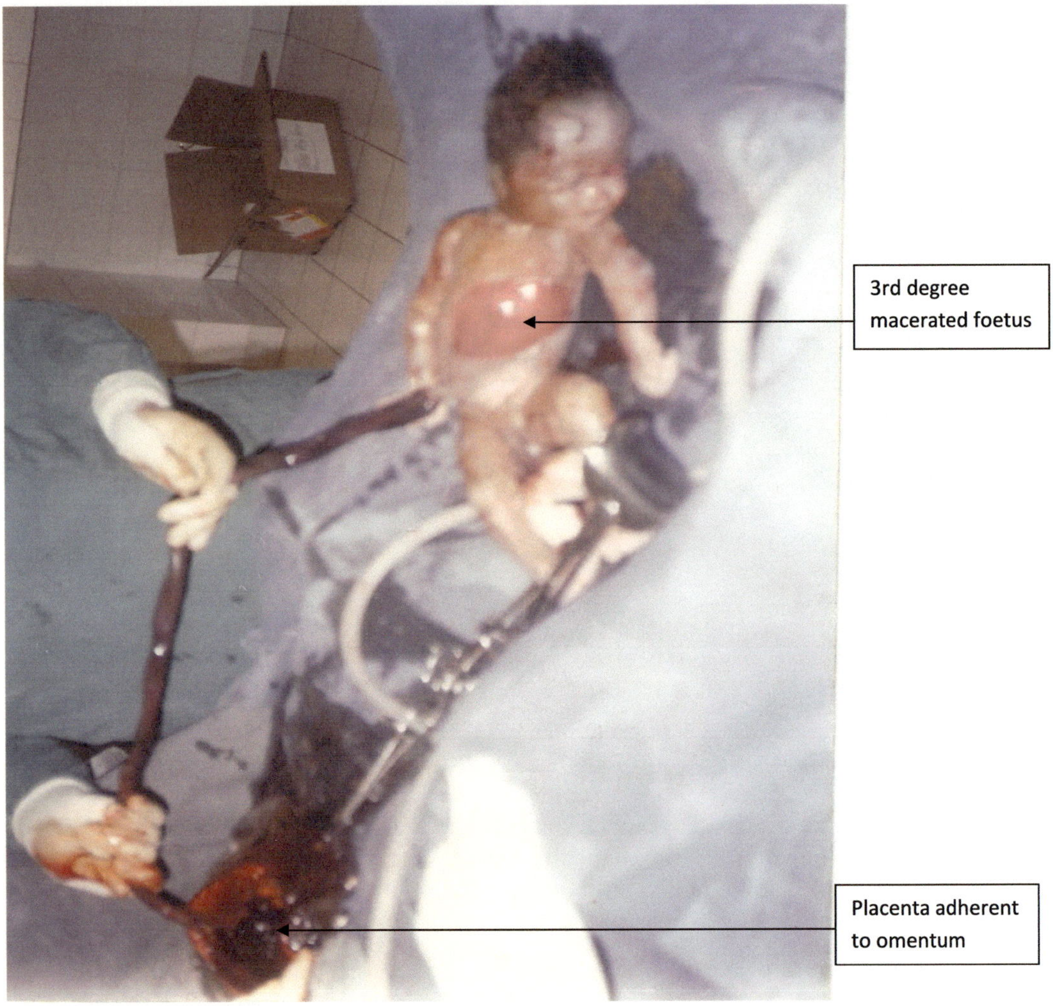

[Dr. Nana's P.N's collection]

Fig. 2. Macerated foetus from perforated uterus.

5.1 Medication abortion

African countries are barely initiating the technique of medication abortion mostly because of the restrictive abortion laws that still prevail. The technique consist of administering Mifeprostone 200mg orally followed by four tablets of prostaglandin (Misoprostol 200 ug), administered vaginally or sublingually 24-48 hours later.

6. Strategies to avoid the tragedy of induced abortions [9,10,14,15,16]

In view of the prevalence of adolescent sexuality, unwanted and unplanned pregnancies, lack of male support and teenage marriages in the developing countries, especially Africa South of the Sahara, it is not surprising that abortion has become a major public health issue. In this respect society today has to take cognizance of the existence of the problem and some strategies to curb and probably avoid the tragedy of induced abortions would include the following:

- **Primary prevention of unsafe abortion:** This means avoiding unwanted and unplanned pregnancy through the following actions:
  - Education of youths: Several studies have shown that education of the girl influences the age of first marriage, intercourse and pregnancy. The tragedy of unwanted teenage pregnancy and the consequences of induced abortions will therefore be reduced. Increased education of the girl also prevents early pregnancy and marriage. Teenage marriage and pregnancy is commoner in communities where the girls do not attain secondary education.
  - Sex Education: This constitutes a component of youth education and must be started at home by parents. Teenage pregnancy is today seen at eleven and twelve years and therefore sex education should start much earlier. In a study published by Leke et al, 38.6% of all induced abortions were carried out by teenagers (10-19 years), and 30% of them were not conversant with their ovulation period. Sex education should be taught to both sexes.
  - Traditional Practices: Some traditional practices are in favour of teenage marriages. Likewise some prohibit pregnancy before marriage or before the education of the girl. Factors like early marriages favour teenage unwanted and unplanned pregnancies, leading to induced abortion and its consequences. In Africa, 20% of all pregnancies occur in the adolescents and 70% of all pregnant adolescents are unmarried or are in union. Adolescent marriage is also a common cause of divorce in Africa. Traditional Doctors are also providers of abortion services, and use quack methods (insertion of cassava stalk or other objects into the cervix). These unfavourable traditional practices must be abolished either by policy makers, chiefs of communities or through the education of the adolescents, parents and the community.
  - Access to Health Services: Provider attitude towards adolescents with unwanted pregnancy may encourage the pregnancy to be carried to term. On the other hand, improper counseling may lead to the desire to terminate the pregnancy.
- **Secondary Prevention:** This involves the provision of abortion service within the context of the law. Post abortion care services should also be made accessible to patients. The introduction of the MVA into all the health structures of the country coupled with training of providers amongst the nurses, midwives and General Practitioners will improve on patient care. The introduction of medication abortion with mifeprostone and misoprostol in the management of missed abortions will also help in the reduction of abortion related complications.
- **Tertiary Prevention:** This entails counseling and the provision of family planning. It is advisable and indicated to start a family planning method before discharge after abortion because ovulation can occur within two weeks of abortion and 75% of the women will be ovulating within six weeks of the abortion. The other reproductive

health services such as cancer screening, infertility, sexually transmitted infection control and nutritional counseling should be considered. The integration of these services ensures better utilization of personnel and service and better sustainability of programmes in low resource areas.

Abortion prevention cannot be limited to health providers alone. The prevention is therefore multi-disciplinary involving several sectors which include:

- Health system: The absence of adolescent clinics in our hospitals is a hindrance to service delivery to this group. Adolescent clinics will permit adolescent needs to be specially addressed.
- Social Welfare Structures: With the economic recession that has hit the nation since the 1990s´, cases of child abandonment and infanticide are seen in our services. Social welfare structures to cater for those babies and their young mothers are nonexistent. Such a service will certainly reduce the rate of abandonment and will favour the reinstatement in schools, thus improving in the health of the adolescent girl.
- Youth Involvement. In all programmes destined for the improvement of the youths it is absolutely necessary to involve the young people themselves in the conception and the implementation of the programme. The community should be consulted and involved, while the community health care provider (Traditional birth attendant) should be trained, provided a limited scope of activity and supervised.
- Review and reinforcement of the abortion law: The economic crisis of the 90´s in some African countries has lead to unemployment and low salaries for health personnel. Health personnel (Doctors and Nurses) are involving themselves more and more in induced abortions as a source of income, almost creating Abortion networks. They may be competent in uterine evacuation techniques but the procedures are carried out under unsafe conditions. Post abortion infection complications and other morbidities do occur to add to the number of abortions carried out by unqualified staff. The abortion law governing safe abortion practice has to be reinforced to prevent such complications and women should be permitted to obtain safe abortion service within the limits of the law. The restricted laws need to be revisited and modified to ease access to safe abortion services.

Complications of unsafe abortion are a major cause of human suffering. In order to address the issue:

Policy makers must examine the factors behind the reliance on unsafe abortion. It is now appropriate for serious discussions to be carried out on the abortion law, develop laws and policies that will reduce mortality and morbidity from unsafe induced abortion. By so doing the health budget as well as individual finances spent in the management of abortion complications will be used in other areas of reproductive health.

Health care Providers can play a major role in the delivery of abortion services through the creation of links by identifying and talking with key actors who often represent the shared interests of the broader communities. These actors include: government officials, leaders of women´s groups, leaders of youth groups, traditional medicine healers, health-committee members, leaders of men´s groups, religious leaders, traditional birth attendants and community-based health worker.

Other activities that can be provided by health care providers are:

- Increase awareness and education by providing women, their families and their partners with needed information on unplanned pregnancy, the availability of contraceptive services, legal indications for induced abortion, dangers of unsafe abortion and the importance of seeking abortion related care only from trained providers.
- Ensure immediate treatment of complications through a comprehensive approach to abortion care. To reduce maternal morbidity and mortality from induced abortion, early counseling and use of family planning is advised. Adequate treatment of abortion complication and correct follow-up will help to reduce morbidity and mortality from induced abortion.
- Monitor service delivery through the creation of quality of-care committees to assist in assessing services, make recommendations and participate in the implementation. Health care providers will also share results of the monitoring process within committee meetings.
- Prevention of infection through the respect of basic hygienic measures in the service and outside the service, especially the disposal of hospital waste materials.
- Advocate for improved policies carried out at grassroots level together with other stakeholders and non-governmental organizations working in the area.

Health care Providers in their mission to reduce maternal mortality and morbidity, a consequence of induced abortion will carry out other activities such as:

- Hands-on training of junior staff and task shifting of abortion care to Midwives and General Practitioners.
- Offering abortion services to the full extent of the law of the country.
- Creating clinics to counsel women on family planning methods and provide family services.
- Using professional bodies to introduce new technologies in abortion care and family planning and to organize training of Trainers courses in comprehensive abortion care.

In order to reduce maternal mortality and morbidity due to unsafe abortion, the following additional measures must be reinforced:

- Ensure immediate post abortion care in unsafe abortion.
- Ensure post abortion family planning service and its extension to risk groups.
- Institute training and counseling of service providers in post abortion care.
- Advocate for modification of the restrictive laws.
- Encourage community participation in the prevention of unsafe abortion.
- Fight for the prioritization of reproductive health programmes.

7. Adolescents and young women

Adolescent Health is one of the eight components of reproductive health. This group of women is still to be properly taken care of within our health institutions. They are seen at consultation with their parents and sometimes this may hinder good communication between the health care provider and the adolescent or young unmarried woman. There is need therefore to create adolescent clinics within our health settings to cater for the problems of the young woman and adolescent. Safe, respectful abortion information and care are essential to ensure young women´s and adolescents´ sexual and reproductive health and well being. Pregnancy and motherhood outside of marriage are stigmatized in many societies, which may cause young, unmarried pregnant women to seek abortion. Other reasons that may favour the decision to terminate a pregnancy in this group are: a desire to continue education, an unsupportive or no partner, inadequate resources, pregnancy resulted from violence or abuse, health risks, or she doesn´t want to become a mother at that time or age.

Unsafe abortion is a large contributor to maternal mortality and morbidity among young women. It has been reported that adolescent girls in developing countries undergo at least 2.2-4 million unsafe abortions each year. In sub- Saharan Africa, over 60% of unsafe abortions are among young women younger than 25 years. Worldwide, young women under the age of 20 make up to 70% of all hospitalizations from unsafe abortion complications. In 2003, young women accounted for approximately 45% of the estimated unsafe-abortion- related deaths. [17] There are many social, economic, logistical, policy and health-system barriers to safe abortion care for young women, these barriers consist of: stigma and negative attitudes, fear of negative repercussions, lack of access to comprehensive sexuality education, limited financial resources, cost of care, transportation, involvement of laws and concerns over privacy and confidentiality. Young women therefore resort to unsafe abortion even in environments where abortion is legal or seek abortion service or treatment for abortion complications much latter than married women [10, 17].

Abortion care service for young women must therefore have the following characteristics:

- Respect for young women and adolescents and their rights.
- Participation by the young women in all stages of service delivery.
- Accessibility.
- Safety and appropriateness.

8. Conclusion

The observed global change in sexual behavior, particularly among the youths is to a large extent responsible for the increased prevalence of unwanted pregnancies and its consequence induced abortion. It must be emphasized that women will continue to seek to terminate unwanted pregnancy by abortion despite the great risk to their health and life. Induced abortion and its complications place a great burden on the limited individual, hospital and community resources, as it often prolongs the duration of hospitalization. The unavailability and inaccessibility of family planning to the semi-urban and rural populations in developing countries explains the high rate of unwanted pregnancies and the complications of induced abortion.

The above statements under conclusion are in line with the conclusion of Konje J.C. and al [18] who ended their studies in Ibadan with the following words «Provision of legal abortion would reduce the incidence of sepsis after termination while reproductive health education and information dissemination and provision of accessible family planning services would greatly reduce the number of unwanted pregnancies" and of course their consequences like induced abortions and complications.

Legal access to abortion services must be accompanied by equipment and commodities at the facilities to offer abortions, by training of providers in modern technology in abortion care as well as availability and easy access to family planning.

9. References

[1] COOK R.J. (1989) Abortion laws and policies challenges and opportunities. International Journal of Obstetrics and Gynecology, Supplement 3. Pp, 61-87.

[2] Royston E, Amstrong S. (eds) (1990) preventing maternal Death, Geneva: WHO Scott, RJ (1986) Spontaneous abortion in obstetrics and gynecology, 3rd edition, D.N Danforth et al. Philadelphis: J, V Lipi Co.

[3] Leke R.J.I, Nana P.N, Halle M.G, Nehemiah K. National Assessment of the magnitude and direct cost of abortion in Cameroon 2009.

[4] Edmonds D.K et al, (1982). Early embryonic mortality in women, Fertility and Sterility, 38, pp. 447-453.

[5] Enquête nationale sur la fécondité au Cameroun (1988) Yaoundé : Ministry of Public Health Cameroon.

[6] Leke R.J.I, Tikum H. (1991). Prospective study of abortion patterns in the Central Maternity, Yaoundé. Vie et Santé 7 pp 8-11.

[7] Kwasi B.F. Kidane-Mariam, W.Saed.E.M. and Forbes, F.G.R (1985) Epidemiology of maternal mortality in Addis Ababa: A community study. Ethiopian Medical Journal, 23 (7), pp.7-16.

[8] Henshaw S.K (1990). Induced abortion: a world review, International family planning perspectives 16, N0 2.

[9] Access to safe abortion (June 2008). International Planned Parenthood Federation.

[10] Hyman, Alyson G, Laura C. 2005. Woman –centered abortion Care: reference manual. Chapel Hill, NC, Ipas.

[11] First Trimester abortion guidelines and protocols. Surgical and medical procedures (September 2008). International Planned Parenthood Federation.

[12] Nana P.N, Fomulu J.N, Mbu R.E, Ako S.N, Leke R.J.I. A four years retrospective review of post Abortal surgical complications of the Central maternity Yaoundé, Cameroon. Clinical mother Child health 2005. Vol 2, No 2: 359-363.

[13] Mbango C. et al, (1987 Reproductive mortality in Lusaka, Zambia, 1982-1983. Studies in family planning, 17(5).pp.243-251.

[14] Leke R.J.I(1990). Approche fondée sur La notion de risque comme stratégies de réduction de la mortalité maternelle: L´expérience de Yaoundé présenté aux congrès de la société gynécologie-obstétrique, Décembre 1990.

[15] Starrs A, (1987) Preventing the tragedy of maternal deaths. A report presented to the International safe Motherhood Conference, Nairobi, Kenya.

[16] Annibal Faundes et Dorothy Shaw: (2010)- Accès universel à la Santé Reproductive : Opportunités pour prévenir les avortements à risque et combler les lacunes critiques en la matière- International Journal Gynéco-obstétrique Vol 110 supplement 1 (2010)

[17] Turner, Katherine L., Evelina B, Amanda H, Cansas M. 2001. Abortion care for young women: A training toolkit. Chapel Hill, NC: Ipas.

[18] Konje J.C, Obisesan K.A, Ladipo O.A(1992).Health and economic consequences of septic induced abortion.Int.J.Gynecol.Obstet.37:193-197

[19] Abortion: A tabulation of available data on the frequency and mortality of unsafe abortion. WHO 1994.
[20] Andrzej K, Malcolm P, Rosenfield A 1996: Abortion and fertility regulation. The Lancet.Vol 347 (1996).

7

The Importance of Urethrocystoscopy and Bladder Biopsy in Gynecologic Patients

Oscar Flores-Carreras, María Isabel González Ruiz, and Claudia Josefina Martínez Espinoza
Urodifem de Occidente, S.C., Mexico

1. Introduction

Some gynecological dysfunctions, but especially the urogynecological ones, require an endoscopic study and in the presence of structural changes, a biopsy.

The main purpose of this chapter is to feel the close relationship between the female genital tract and the lower urinary tract (LUT) that leads to clinical dysfunctions that can impact either one and cause symptoms with increased severity or significance than the initially affected. A representative example of this would be the Painful Urethral Syndrome, which can cause severe dyspareunia that affects in a significant degree the couple's relationship. In the pelvic compartment, pelvic organ prolapse may cause symptoms of the lower urinary tract both in the filling and emptying phases. In many of these diseases the study of the lower urinary tract symptoms (LUTS) makes it necessary to evaluate the urethra and bladder endoscopically and perform a biopsy when an organic disease is found.

This chapter will focus on those conditions, that according to our experience justifies the expressed above.

1.1 Historical perspective

The practice of bladder biopsy is intimately related to the history of urethrocystoscopy that Puigvert narrated(1939). Bozzini in 1805 described the first cystoscope consisting of a metal tube which on the extravesical end applied a spark plug through which the visual field was illuminated and limited at the other end of the tube. Then Desormeaux (1853) submitted to the Paris Academy of Medicine a cystoscope made by him, which consisted of the urethral tube and a lighting apparatus provider of a lamp which burnt a mixture of alcohol and turpentine, whose light reflected, by mirror lit by the tube, the bladder´s cavity. Thirteen years later he published the first book on the subject "Treaty of Urinary Endoscopy and its Applications to the Diagnosis and Treatment of Urethrovesical Conditions". In 1886, Max Nitze built a cystoscope with an optical system almost identical to that used today, equipped with an incandescent Edison lighting system.

Howard A. Kelly was appointed the first professor of gynecology at the John Hopkins Medical School. Kelly (1893) believed that gynecology and urology were so closely related that one could not be trained in either field and ignore the other. Kelly invented in 1914 the urethroscope and emphasized the importance to explore endoscopically not only the bladder but also and principally the female urethra.

Jack R. Robertson (1973) returned to Kelly´s concepts and applied modern technology updating Kelly´s urethroscope by providing it with a gas source and a recording equipment, calling it "Gynecologic urethroscope". Robertson emphasized the dynamic study of the urethra, asking the patient to strain, contract the pelvic floor and to cough, in order to assess the neuromuscular physiological response.

His concepts, strictly followed by us, strongly influenced the International gynecological environment which favored the creation of the American Urogynecological Society. Robertson was its first President in 1979.

Suprapubic telescopy described by Timmons (1990), has been a significant progress. He placed special emphasis in the intraoperative diagnosis of ureteral injury, assessing the elimination of indigo carmine through the ureteral meatus after the introduction of the cystoscope through a small hole in the extraperitoneal bladder wall.

Interestingly a variant of suprapubic teloscopy was already practiced by French urologists (1920), under the title "hypogastric cystoscopy", among them Kraske, who used a special cystoscope equipped with a tip ending in a sharp point. The technique was refined by Katz and Kolisher who performed a suprapubic fistula and used the ordinary cystoscope.

Endoscopy of the LUT in women has been a remarkable progress for the gynecologist and for the development of Urogynecology.

2. Bladder biopsy

The first bladder biopsy forceps were independently described by Young and Marion in1929, by which it was possible to extract portions of tumor tissue, according to the description of Puigvert (1939).

Currently the general criterion is to perform a bladder biopsy when there is tumor formation or epithelial change that may represent suspicious malignant lesions. In cases where there is no tumor but an epithelial disruption exists, the indication of biopsy is priority if a urinary cytology is positive.

Bladder cancers are classified as being non-muscle-invasive or muscle invasive according to their histological appearance. Non-muscle-invasive bladder cancers account for about 70 to 80% of all bladder cancers (Abel 1988; VanDer Meijde et al. 1999). The primary approach for Ta and T1 tumors is transurethral resection of bladder tumor. The main problem after the initial treatment of non-muscle-invasive cancers is the high recurrence rate (40 to 80%) Gogus et al.(2002). Many prognostic factors, such as tumor stage, tumor grade, multiplicity, concomitant carcinoma in situ and tumor size have been proposed to affect tumor recurrence of non-muscle-invasive bladder carcinoma (May et al. 2003) (Kiemeney et al. (1994).

Additionally, bladder biopsy is also used in patients previously treated for bladder cancer as a method of detection and control. In these cases the criteria for performing biopsy include suspicious lesions or areas of red urothelium (Lee et al. 2009), but some authors advocate biopsy even in the absence of epithelial disruption. This approach is controversial and it is not in accordance with international guidelines (Matsuchima et al. 2010).

The indication of cystoscopy is controversial. If the object is only the detection of neoplasms of the LUT, a generalized concept is to practice it in the presence of macro or microscopic hematuria or in the presence of a positive urinary cytology with cells suspicious of malignancy. Nevertheless, microscopic hematuria is not a predictive factor for cancer, several authors confirm this. Wu et al. (2006) of 735 patients with irritative symptoms, only 35.9% of the cancers had hematuria. Goldberg et al. (2008) reported that only 40% of cancer patients present hematuria. Flores-Carreras et al. (2010) evaluated 331 women with LUTS of which 62.8% had symptoms of overactive bladder and 31.4% had hematuria. Bladder cancer was diagnosed in two cases (0.6%), similar percentage than that reported by others authors, (0.2% to 3.9%) (Lee et al. 2009; Borden et al. 2003; Sokol et al. 2005). None of the cancer cases had hematuria. They also detected three cases of Cystitis Glandularis of which two had no history of hematuria and two cases of papillomatous tumor, both positive for hematuria. The clinical morphologic and hystopathologic diagnosis is showed in Table1.

Diagnosis	with hematuria		without hematuria	
	N	%	N	%
INTERSTITIAL CYSTITIS	5	14.3	10	28.6
BLADDER PAPILLOMA	2	5.7	----	----
CHRONIC CYSTITIS	1	2.9	3	8.6
CYSTITIS FOLLICULARIS	1	2.9	3	8.6
BLADDER CANCER	-----	-----	1	2.9
CYSTITIS GLANDULARIS	1	2.9	2	5.7
ACUTE CYSTITIS	----	----	1	2.9
ANGIOMATOSE POLYP	----	----	1	2.9
POLIPOID CYSTITIS	----	----	1	2.9
MICROPAPILLOMATOSIS	----	-----	1	2.9
IN SITU BLADDER CANCER			1	2.9
SQUAMOUS METAPLASIA			1	2.9
TOTAL	10	28.6	25	71.4

Table 1. Clinical, morphologic and histopathology diagnosis in 35 bladder biopsies. Comparative results in patients with and without hematuria.

It is a comparative pathologic result between hematuria and not hematuria cases. As it is possible to see, the most frequent diagnosis was Interstitial Cystitis in both groups (42.9%) of the total cases.

Smoking has been considered a major risk factor for bladder cancer and is responsible for almost half the deaths from bladder cancer in men (48%), and less than a third among women (Pashos et al. 2002). This was the reason why we investigated it and were able to detect 10 patients who smoked (28.6%). One of the two bladder cancer patients was a smoker.

2.1 Background

A characteristic of urogynecologic patients with regards to their symptoms is that such symptoms are non-specific. Thus one commonly sees symptoms in patients with stress or urge incontinence similar to the ones in patients with a local irritation due to infection, distal stenosis or a neoplastic process.

2.2 Technique

For the urethrocystoscopy, patients were placed in lithotomy position, followed by cleansing the introitus with an antiseptic solution. The order of the endoscopy is to start with the urethroscopy followed by the cystoscopy. For distention in both cases sterile saline solution at room temperature is used.

For the urethroscopy we use the Robertson monitor which is proved for a 0-degree telescope and as mentioned before, perform the dynamic urethroscopy and also visualize the color, the presence of inflammatory signs or any structural lesion as stenosis, fistula or diverticulum. Our particular point of view is that urethroscopy is the best and most practical diagnostic method to detect the presence of diverticulum and obviously, of urethral tumors and urethritis. For the cystoscopy, we use Karl Storz 70° lenses with a 18Fr sheath for exploring, or 22Fr sheath in case of operatory endoscopy. In case of biopsy, flexible 7Fr caliber forceps (Karl Storz) are used. For distention in both cases we used sterile saline solution at room temperature.

In the first ten biopsies we applied xylocaine gel as a local anesthetic, but when the product disappeared from the local market, the biopsy on the rest of the patients was performed without anesthesia. This procedure is well tolerated by the patient if we previously inform of it. This procedure is carried out in the office with the inherent advantages this entails, in terms of the risks and financial expenses brought about by a hospital procedure (Flores Carreras et al. 2010).

2.3 Overviewing

There are many pelvic conditions that affect the LUT: chronic pelvic pain, pelvic organ prolapse, postmenopausal hormonal deprivation, vulvar-vaginal infectious processes, lesions of the LUT and pelvic surgery for benign and malignant tumors of the female genital tract. Also urinary problems that affect the gynecological function and well being for example: urinary incontinence, voiding dysfunction, postoperative vulvar-vaginal stenosis, overactive bladder, urethral pain syndrome, Bladder Pain Syndrome/Interstitial Cystitis

(BPS/IC). In some of these conditions, bladder biopsy is advisable; in this chapter we'll discuss pros and cons of this procedure.

Specialized medical literature contains conflicting positions regarding the systematic use of urethrocystoscopy in female patients with LUTS. There are those who recommend the procedure (Lee et al. 2009; Goldberg et al 2008; Cundiff & Bent 1996) and others who restrict it to patients with irritability symptoms together with macro or micro hematuria. In any event, the general consensus is to consider urethral cystoscopy the "gold standard" method to diagnose bladder cancer (Abel 1988; VanDer Meijde et al. 1999). In our opinion, we must incorporate urethrocystoscopy into our protocol to examine patients suffering from: 1) mixed urinary incontinence, 2) hyperactive bladder, 3) macro or micro hematuria, 4) bladder or pelvic pain related with LUTS, 5) recurrent urinary tract infection, 6) urinary symptoms related with pelvic surgery, 7) bladder or urethral tenderness, 8) during pelvic surgery to exclude bladder or ureteral lesion.

About the different points of view Lee et al. (2009) expressed the following concepts: "There are many different points of view related to the practice of cystoscopy between urologists and urogynecologists. For the first one, hematuria is the single most common indication; in contrast, urogynecologists not only perform cystoscopy but also urethroscopy and they visualize the lower urinary tract more thoroughly for a broad range of indications, most commonly for exclusion of intravesical lesions in women with LUTS or recurrent urinary tract infection (RUTI), suspected foreign body and diagnosis of urethral diverticulum".

2.4 Urinary incontinence

In this chapter our position is to practice urethrocystoscopy in patients who accuse mixed incontinence (stress and urgency), recurrent or continuous or pure urgency. It is not necessary an endoscopic study of patients with only stress incontinence, not previously treated surgically, and when bladder neck prolapse is demonstrated. It is especially important to perform endoscopic evaluation in patients with recurrent incontinence because you can find in them, a number of surgical sequels of injury of pelvic structures whose non-detection should be classified as a professional negligence. Continuous incontinence mostly preceded by surgery and urgency incontinence, usually accompanied by symptoms of bladder irritability, requires endoscopic study, from our point of view.

2.5 Overactive bladder

The International Continence Society (Abrams et al. 2002) defines the overactive bladder (OAB) as "urgency, with or without urge incontinence, usually with frequency and nocturia…if there is not proven infection or other etiology."

The overall prevalence of OAB in United States was 16.9% in women and 16.0% in men, increasing with age. The overall prevalence of OAB dry and OAB wet was 7.6% and 9.3% in women respectively, and 13.6% and 2.6% respectively in men (Noble Program) (Stewart et al. 2003). Although the prevalence of this condition increases with advancing age, having overactive bladder is abnormal at any age. Overall, it is estimated that 17% of the general population over 40 years of age suffers from overactive bladder. Similar prevalence is reported in Europe.

The cause of OAB is unknown in the vast majority of patients. In a few rare cases, it may develop secondary to neurologic disorders, such as stroke, multiple sclerosis or spinal cord injuries. Other causes have been described such as: bladder outlet obstruction, pelvic organ prolapse, impaired detrusor contraction, diabetes, between others. Shaw et al., and Ikeda et al., have reported as risk factors: Caucasian race, insulin-dependent diabetes, alcohol intake and history of depression (Shaw et al. 2011; Ikeda et al. 2011).

Most authors recommend basic evaluations that consist of a focused history and examination, bladder diary and urinalysis. A more detailed diagnostic evaluation is only recommended after treatment failure, if there is micro hematuria or elevated residual urine.

From our point of view, we should perform, in addition to medical history, urinary diary, urine culture, uroflowmetry, investigation of residual urine and urethrocystoscopy. This attitude, which might be considered radical for some physicians, represents for us a complete and secure exploratory approach. Detection of the above-mentioned four tumors would not been possible with a more conservative behavior.

2.6 Chronic pelvic pain

Chronic pelvic pain is a typical example of possible indication of endoscopic study of the LUT, especially when the pain is topographically expressed in the suprapubic region, vaginal canal or vulvar area and/or accompanied by urinary increased disorders such as frequency, nocturia and urgency.

The typical bladder pain is felt suprapubically and generally increases with bladder filling and may persist after voiding. Painful bladder syndrome is defined by the International Continence Society (ICS) as suprapubic pain that is related to bladder filling in the absence of proven urinary tract disorders such as infection or other pathology and is often associated with increased frequency and nocturia (Abrams et al. 2002).

Painful bladder syndrome is frequently associated with Interstitial Cystitis that is why denomination PBS/IC was established by the ICS.

The exact prevalence of Painful Bladder Syndrome/Interstitial Cystitis is unknown. Clemens et al., (2005) estimated that in United States of America, one million people suffer IC of which 90% are women. In the last 20 years several epidemiological studies have noted an increase in frequency with values of 25.1, 36.6, 76.3, per 100,000 habitants (Curhan et al. 1999). A relatively recent study reported a prevalence of 0.51% in USA (Jone et al. 1994). In our private urogynecology unit (Urodifem de Occidente S.C.) of a total of 331 female patients studied, the diagnosis of BPS/IC was established in 18 cases (3/15) (Flores Carreras et al. 2010), representing a rate of 5.4% for a unit specializing in urogynecology problems. Biopsy was taken in 14 cases and their histological finding was consistent with those described for IC: lymphoplasmacytic infiltration, fibrosis reaction and in some cases, increase in the number of mast cells. In any case were noted signs of malignancy. The thirty-three of patients with BPS/IC had hematuria.

2.7 Urethral painful syndrome

The urethral painful syndrome (UPS) is a condition very common in women. In some patients the onset is at an early age even in nubile women with "nonbacterial cystitis" expressed in dehydrated patients or coinciding with menses. Often the first expression of this condition is the initiation of sexual activity and therefore has acquired the name of "honeymoon cystitis".

In 2002 the I.C.S defined it as "Occurrence of persistent or recurrent episodic of urethral pain usually on voiding with daytime frequency and nocturia in the absence of proven infection or other obvious pathology". The diagnosis implies longevity symptoms of at least 6 months of duration. The incidence and prevalence of this condition is not known due to the lack of consensus about this condition. Some authors have reported that 15-30% of women who presented with lower urinary tract symptoms were diagnosed as urethral pain syndrome. The prevalence in our casuistic was of 31.4%.

This condition is usually inflammatory in nature. Frequently there are lumps of pus through the periurethral glands seen at urethroscopy, especially when simultaneous urethral massage is performed, however microbiological studies are generally negative. We feel that urethroscopy is very important in these cases to confirm the state of inflammation of the urethra and to detect underlying pathology such as a narrow meatus, urethral diverticulum, suburethral cyst, among other conditions. Many of these patients have been treated with antibiotics with poor results.

In our experience UPS is one of the conditions that mostly affects the couple´s sexual identification because it causes dyspareunia or vulvar-vaginal pain after intercourse and occur during the beginning of sexual life. Management is difficult, based on antimicrobial, urethral dilatations, urethral massage, anti-cholinergics, anti-inflammatory drugs, smooth muscle relaxants, precoital lubricants and even emotional and technical support to the couple. We should always rule out the presence of chlamydia and ureaplasma.

2.8 Recurrent urinary tract infection (RUTI)

For definitional purposes RUTI refers to more than three infections in one year (Nickel et al. 1991). The current incidence of urinary infection among premenopausal, sexual active women is 0.5-0.7 infections/person year. Furthermore, 20% of women will have a urinary tract infection (UTI) in their lifetime with 3% having RUTI. Recurrent infections are due to either reinfection or bacterial persistent. Reinfection is recurrent infection with different bacteria. The majority of infections are asymptomatic and clear spontaneously (Lawrentschuk et al. 2006). In symptomatic patients the most common symptoms are dysuria, frequency, urgency, nocturia and suprapubic discomfort. Occasionally mild incontinence and hematuria may occur.

Gram-negative bacilli of the family Enterobacteriaceae are responsible for 90% of infections. E. Coli is the single most important organism and accounts for 80 to 90% of uncomplicated infections.

The value of routine cystoscopy investigation has not been clearly defined; there are different opinions such as Fowler and Pulanski (1981), who noted that in young patients the only abnormality that altered treatment was a urethral diverticulum. However, the published literature is in favor of cystoscopy in women with RUTI, principally in patients of more than 50 years old (Lawrentschuk et al. 2006; Van Haarst et al. 2001).

There are certain risk factors for developing urinary infections: hematuria, pyelonefritis, calculi, diabetes, in the elderly patients, urethral obstruction, pelvic surgery and urethral diverticulum (Lawrentschuk et al. 2006). The majority of urinary tract infections are ascending infections from the fecal flora which colonize the vaginal introitus, then the periurethral tissues, and eventually gain entry to the bladder.

3. Conclusions

Urethrocystoscopy and eventual bladder biopsy are an integral tool for the evaluation of lower urinary tract symptoms, to make possible the detection of structural lesions, benign or malignant tumors and exclude injuries of the urinary tract between other problems. Almost all of the urogynecologists support the indication of urethrocystoscopy in patients with dysfunction of the lower urinary tract. Urethrocystoscopy provides an anatomical assessment of the urethra and bladder that is not accomplished with urodynamics or other types of tests. If we think only in order of detection of malignant tumors, younger women (less than 50 years) are less likely to have pathology; this condition must be factored into decision to perform or not endoscopy. However, bladder cancer is an important reason to keep in mind for women with abnormal voiding symptoms even in the presence of a normal urinalysis. The rate of detection of cancer in women with LUTS goes from 0.2 to 3.9% (in our casuistic 0.6%). The majority of the cases were discovered in patients presenting without hematuria.

Finally, we consider that a physician who treats women with lower urinary tract symptoms is obligated to provide reasonable assurance that the patient's urinary system is otherwise normal.

4. References

Abel PD. Prognostic indices in transitional cell carcinoma of the bladder Br. J. Urol. 1988;62:103-109.

Abrams P, Cardozo L, Fall M et al. The Standardization of terminology of lower urinary tract function: Report from the standardization subcommittee of the international continence society. Neurourol. Urodyn. 2002;21:167-78.

Borden LS Jr.,Clarck PE, Hall MC. Bladder cancer. Curr. Opinion Oncol. 2003;15:227-33

Clemens JQ, Meenan RT, Rosetti MC, Calhoun EA. Prevalence e incidence of I.C. in a managed care population. J. Urol. 2005;173:98-102.

Cundiff JW, Bent AE. The contribution of urethrocystoscopy to evaluation of lower urinary tract dysfunction in women. Int. Urogynecol. J. 1996;7:307-311.

Curhan GC, Speizer FE, Hunter DJ. Et al. Epidemiology of interstitial cystitis: a population based study. J. Urol. 1999;161:549-

Flores Carreras O, Gonzalez RI, Martinez EC., Montes C. Y. a) Contribución de la biopsia vesical al estudio de la paciente uroginecológica. Ginecol. Obstet. Mex. 2010;78(3):187-190. b) Evaluación clínica y diagnostica en pacientes con Cistitis Intersticial. Ginecol. Obstet. Mex. 2010;78(5):275-280.

Fowler JE, Pulanski ET. Urography, cystography and cystoscopy in women with urinary tract infection. N. England J. Med. 1981;304:462-5

Gogus C, Bodur Y, Turcolines K, Gogus O. The significance of random bladder biopsies in superficial bladder cancer. Int. Urol. Nephrol. 2002;34:59-61.

Goldberg JM, Sherman W, Sand PK. Cystoscopy for lower urinary tract symptoms in urogynecologic practice. The likelihood of finding bladder cancer. Int. Uroginecol. J. 2008;19:991-994.

Ikeda Y, Haruo I, Ohmorj M, Hosawa A, Masamure Y, Nishino Y, Kuriyama S, Ohnuma T, Tsuji I, Aral Y. Int. J. of Urology 2011;18(3):212-218.

Jone CA, Harris M, Nyberg L. Prevalence of Cystitis Interstitial in the United States J. Urol. 1994;151:423A.

Kelly H.A. Bull of Johns Hopkins Hospital. November 1893.

Kiemeney LA, Witjes JA, Heigbrock RP, Debruyne FM, Verbeek AL. Dysplasia in normal-looking urothelium increases the risk of tumor progression in primary superficial bladder cancer. Eur. J. Cancer 1994;30A:1621-1625.

Lawrentschuk N, Jason OOI, Pang A, Krishant SN and Bolton DM. Cystoscopy in women with recurrent urinary tract infection. Int. J. of Urology.2006:13:350-353-

Lee JWS, Dowmouchtis SK, Jeffery S, Fynes MM. Evaluation of outpatient cystoscopy in urogynecology. Arch. Gynecol. Obstet. 2009;279: 631-635.

Matsuchima M, Kiguchi E, Hasgagwa M, Matsumoto K, Miyajiwua A, Oya M. Clinical impact of bladder biopsies with TUR-BT according to cytology results in patient with bladder cancer: a case control study. Urol. 2010;10:12-15.

May F, Treiber V, Hartang R, Schaibold H. Significance of random bladder biopsies in superficial bladder cancer. Eur. Urol. 2003;44:47-50.

Nickel JC, Wilson J, Morales A, Heaton J. Value of urologic investigation in a targeted group of women with recurrent urinary tract infection. Can. J. Surg. 1991:34:591-4.

Pashos CL, Botteman MF, LaskinBL, Redaeli A. Bladder cancer epidemiology, diagnosis and management. Cancer Pract. 2002;10: 311-322.

Puigvert A. a) Historia de la endoscopia urinaria. In Puigvert ed. Endoscopia urinaria Barcelona Salvat Eds. S.A 1939;I:14. b)Tumores vesicales In Puigvert ed. Endoscopia urinaria. Barcelona. Salvat Eds. S.A. 1939;XVIII:117-131.

Robertson J.R. Gynecologic urethroscopy. Amer. J. Obstet. Gynecol. 1973;115:986-89.

Shaw H, Burrows MBA, Lara J. Southern Medical J. 2011; 104(1):34-39.

Sokol ER, Patel SR, Sung VW, Randing CR, Watzen S. Clemons JL. Results of Urine Cytology Testing and Cystoscopy in women with irritative Symptoms. Amer. J. Obstet. Gynecol. 2005;192:1560-5.

Stewart W, Payne C, Herzog R, Norton P. Reliability of reporting on symptoms and features of overactive bladder in a community sample . World J. Urol 2003;20:327

Timmons MC. Adisson WA. Suprapubic telescopy extraperitoneal intraoperative technique to demonstrate uretheral patency. Obstet. Gynecol. 1990;75:137-139.

Van Haarst EP, van Andel G, Heldeweg EA, Shlatmann TJ, van der Horst HJ. Evaluation of the diagnostic workup in young women referred for recurrent lower urinary tract infections. Urology 2001;57:1068-72.

Vander Meijden A, Oosterlinck W, Brausi M, Kurth KH, Sylvester R, De Balincourt C; Significance of bladder biopsies inTa,T1 bladder tumors: A report from the

EORTC Genitourinary Tract Cancers Cooperative Group. Eur. Urol. 1999; 35:267-271.

Wu JM, Williams KS, Williams BA, Hundley AF, Jaunelli ML, Visco AG. Microscopic hematuria as predictive factor for detecting bladder cancer at cystoscopy in women with irritative voiding symptoms Amer. J of Obstet. Gynecol. 2006;194:1423-6